Diabetes Log Book

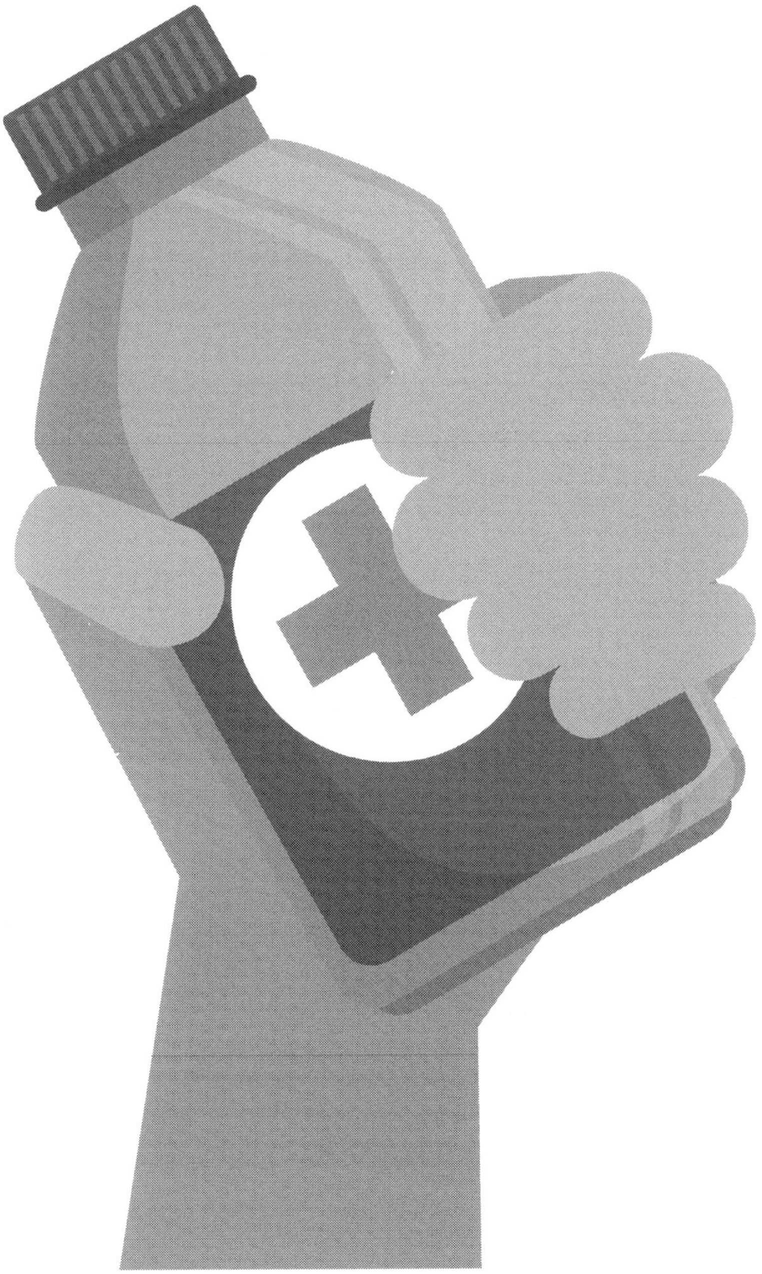

Weekly Diabetes Record

Name: ______________________________

Date:	Breakfast	Snack	Lunch	Snack	Dinner	Snack	Bedtime	Night	Notes
Blood Sugar									
Insulin Dose									
Grams Carb									
Activity									

Date:	Breakfast	Snack	Lunch	Snack	Dinner	Snack	Bedtime	Night	Notes
Blood Sugar									
Insulin Dose									
Grams Carb									
Activity									

Date:	Breakfast	Snack	Lunch	Snack	Dinner	Snack	Bedtime	Night	Notes
Blood Sugar									
Insulin Dose									
Grams Carb									
Activity									

Date:	Breakfast	Snack	Lunch	Snack	Dinner	Snack	Bedtime	Night	Notes
Blood Sugar									
Insulin Dose									
Grams Carb									
Activity									

Date:	Breakfast	Snack	Lunch	Snack	Dinner	Snack	Bedtime	Night	Notes
Blood Sugar									
Insulin Dose									
Grams Carb									
Activity									

Date:	Breakfast	Snack	Lunch	Snack	Dinner	Snack	Bedtime	Night	Notes
Blood Sugar									
Insulin Dose									
Grams Carb									
Activity									

Date:	Breakfast	Snack	Lunch	Snack	Dinner	Snack	Bedtime	Night	Notes
Blood Sugar									
Insulin Dose									
Grams Carb									
Activity									

Weekly Diabetes Record

Name: ______________________________

Date:	Breakfast	Snack	Lunch	Snack	Dinner	Snack	Bedtime	Night	Notes
Blood Sugar									
Insulin Dose									
Grams Carb									
Activity									

Date:	Breakfast	Snack	Lunch	Snack	Dinner	Snack	Bedtime	Night	Notes
Blood Sugar									
Insulin Dose									
Grams Carb									
Activity									

Date:	Breakfast	Snack	Lunch	Snack	Dinner	Snack	Bedtime	Night	Notes
Blood Sugar									
Insulin Dose									
Grams Carb									
Activity									

Date:	Breakfast	Snack	Lunch	Snack	Dinner	Snack	Bedtime	Night	Notes
Blood Sugar									
Insulin Dose									
Grams Carb									
Activity									

Date:	Breakfast	Snack	Lunch	Snack	Dinner	Snack	Bedtime	Night	Notes
Blood Sugar									
Insulin Dose									
Grams Carb									
Activity									

Date:	Breakfast	Snack	Lunch	Snack	Dinner	Snack	Bedtime	Night	Notes
Blood Sugar									
Insulin Dose									
Grams Carb									
Activity									

Date:	Breakfast	Snack	Lunch	Snack	Dinner	Snack	Bedtime	Night	Notes
Blood Sugar									
Insulin Dose									
Grams Carb									
Activity									

Weekly Diabetes Record

Name: ______________________________

Date:	Breakfast	Snack	Lunch	Snack	Dinner	Snack	Bedtime	Night	Notes
Blood Sugar									
Insulin Dose									
Grams Carb									
Activity									

Date:	Breakfast	Snack	Lunch	Snack	Dinner	Snack	Bedtime	Night	Notes
Blood Sugar									
Insulin Dose									
Grams Carb									
Activity									

Date:	Breakfast	Snack	Lunch	Snack	Dinner	Snack	Bedtime	Night	Notes
Blood Sugar									
Insulin Dose									
Grams Carb									
Activity									

Date:	Breakfast	Snack	Lunch	Snack	Dinner	Snack	Bedtime	Night	Notes
Blood Sugar									
Insulin Dose									
Grams Carb									
Activity									

Date:	Breakfast	Snack	Lunch	Snack	Dinner	Snack	Bedtime	Night	Notes
Blood Sugar									
Insulin Dose									
Grams Carb									
Activity									

Date:	Breakfast	Snack	Lunch	Snack	Dinner	Snack	Bedtime	Night	Notes
Blood Sugar									
Insulin Dose									
Grams Carb									
Activity									

Date:	Breakfast	Snack	Lunch	Snack	Dinner	Snack	Bedtime	Night	Notes
Blood Sugar									
Insulin Dose									
Grams Carb									
Activity									

Weekly Diabetes Record

Name: ______________________________

Date:	Breakfast	Snack	Lunch	Snack	Dinner	Snack	Bedtime	Night	Notes
Blood Sugar									
Insulin Dose									
Grams Carb									
Activity									

Date:	Breakfast	Snack	Lunch	Snack	Dinner	Snack	Bedtime	Night	Notes
Blood Sugar									
Insulin Dose									
Grams Carb									
Activity									

Date:	Breakfast	Snack	Lunch	Snack	Dinner	Snack	Bedtime	Night	Notes
Blood Sugar									
Insulin Dose									
Grams Carb									
Activity									

Date:	Breakfast	Snack	Lunch	Snack	Dinner	Snack	Bedtime	Night	Notes
Blood Sugar									
Insulin Dose									
Grams Carb									
Activity									

Date:	Breakfast	Snack	Lunch	Snack	Dinner	Snack	Bedtime	Night	Notes
Blood Sugar									
Insulin Dose									
Grams Carb									
Activity									

Date:	Breakfast	Snack	Lunch	Snack	Dinner	Snack	Bedtime	Night	Notes
Blood Sugar									
Insulin Dose									
Grams Carb									
Activity									

Date:	Breakfast	Snack	Lunch	Snack	Dinner	Snack	Bedtime	Night	Notes
Blood Sugar									
Insulin Dose									
Grams Carb									
Activity									

Weekly Diabetes Record

Name: ______________________________

Date:	Breakfast	Snack	Lunch	Snack	Dinner	Snack	Bedtime	Night	Notes
Blood Sugar									
Insulin Dose									
Grams Carb									
Activity									

Date:	Breakfast	Snack	Lunch	Snack	Dinner	Snack	Bedtime	Night	Notes
Blood Sugar									
Insulin Dose									
Grams Carb									
Activity									

Date:	Breakfast	Snack	Lunch	Snack	Dinner	Snack	Bedtime	Night	Notes
Blood Sugar									
Insulin Dose									
Grams Carb									
Activity									

Date:	Breakfast	Snack	Lunch	Snack	Dinner	Snack	Bedtime	Night	Notes
Blood Sugar									
Insulin Dose									
Grams Carb									
Activity									

Date:	Breakfast	Snack	Lunch	Snack	Dinner	Snack	Bedtime	Night	Notes
Blood Sugar									
Insulin Dose									
Grams Carb									
Activity									

Date:	Breakfast	Snack	Lunch	Snack	Dinner	Snack	Bedtime	Night	Notes
Blood Sugar									
Insulin Dose									
Grams Carb									
Activity									

Date:	Breakfast	Snack	Lunch	Snack	Dinner	Snack	Bedtime	Night	Notes
Blood Sugar									
Insulin Dose									
Grams Carb									
Activity									

Weekly Diabetes Record

Name: ____

Date:	Breakfast	Snack	Lunch	Snack	Dinner	Snack	Bedtime	Night	Notes
Blood Sugar									
Insulin Dose									
Grams Carb									
Activity									

Date:	Breakfast	Snack	Lunch	Snack	Dinner	Snack	Bedtime	Night	Notes
Blood Sugar									
Insulin Dose									
Grams Carb									
Activity									

Date:	Breakfast	Snack	Lunch	Snack	Dinner	Snack	Bedtime	Night	Notes
Blood Sugar									
Insulin Dose									
Grams Carb									
Activity									

Date:	Breakfast	Snack	Lunch	Snack	Dinner	Snack	Bedtime	Night	Notes
Blood Sugar									
Insulin Dose									
Grams Carb									
Activity									

Date:	Breakfast	Snack	Lunch	Snack	Dinner	Snack	Bedtime	Night	Notes
Blood Sugar									
Insulin Dose									
Grams Carb									
Activity									

Date:	Breakfast	Snack	Lunch	Snack	Dinner	Snack	Bedtime	Night	Notes
Blood Sugar									
Insulin Dose									
Grams Carb									
Activity									

Date:	Breakfast	Snack	Lunch	Snack	Dinner	Snack	Bedtime	Night	Notes
Blood Sugar									
Insulin Dose									
Grams Carb									
Activity									

Weekly Diabetes Record

Name: ______________________________

Date:	Breakfast	Snack	Lunch	Snack	Dinner	Snack	Bedtime	Night	Notes
Blood Sugar									
Insulin Dose									
Grams Carb									
Activity									

Date:	Breakfast	Snack	Lunch	Snack	Dinner	Snack	Bedtime	Night	Notes
Blood Sugar									
Insulin Dose									
Grams Carb									
Activity									

Date:	Breakfast	Snack	Lunch	Snack	Dinner	Snack	Bedtime	Night	Notes
Blood Sugar									
Insulin Dose									
Grams Carb									
Activity									

Date:	Breakfast	Snack	Lunch	Snack	Dinner	Snack	Bedtime	Night	Notes
Blood Sugar									
Insulin Dose									
Grams Carb									
Activity									

Date:	Breakfast	Snack	Lunch	Snack	Dinner	Snack	Bedtime	Night	Notes
Blood Sugar									
Insulin Dose									
Grams Carb									
Activity									

Date:	Breakfast	Snack	Lunch	Snack	Dinner	Snack	Bedtime	Night	Notes
Blood Sugar									
Insulin Dose									
Grams Carb									
Activity									

Date:	Breakfast	Snack	Lunch	Snack	Dinner	Snack	Bedtime	Night	Notes
Blood Sugar									
Insulin Dose									
Grams Carb									
Activity									

Weekly Diabetes Record

Name: ______________________________

Date:	Breakfast	Snack	Lunch	Snack	Dinner	Snack	Bedtime	Night	Notes
Blood Sugar									
Insulin Dose									
Grams Carb									
Activity									

Date:	Breakfast	Snack	Lunch	Snack	Dinner	Snack	Bedtime	Night	Notes
Blood Sugar									
Insulin Dose									
Grams Carb									
Activity									

Date:	Breakfast	Snack	Lunch	Snack	Dinner	Snack	Bedtime	Night	Notes
Blood Sugar									
Insulin Dose									
Grams Carb									
Activity									

Date:	Breakfast	Snack	Lunch	Snack	Dinner	Snack	Bedtime	Night	Notes
Blood Sugar									
Insulin Dose									
Grams Carb									
Activity									

Date:	Breakfast	Snack	Lunch	Snack	Dinner	Snack	Bedtime	Night	Notes
Blood Sugar									
Insulin Dose									
Grams Carb									
Activity									

Date:	Breakfast	Snack	Lunch	Snack	Dinner	Snack	Bedtime	Night	Notes
Blood Sugar									
Insulin Dose									
Grams Carb									
Activity									

Date:	Breakfast	Snack	Lunch	Snack	Dinner	Snack	Bedtime	Night	Notes
Blood Sugar									
Insulin Dose									
Grams Carb									
Activity									

Weekly Diabetes Record

Name: ______________________________

Date:	Breakfast	Snack	Lunch	Snack	Dinner	Snack	Bedtime	Night	Notes
Blood Sugar									
Insulin Dose									
Grams Carb									
Activity									

Date:	Breakfast	Snack	Lunch	Snack	Dinner	Snack	Bedtime	Night	Notes
Blood Sugar									
Insulin Dose									
Grams Carb									
Activity									

Date:	Breakfast	Snack	Lunch	Snack	Dinner	Snack	Bedtime	Night	Notes
Blood Sugar									
Insulin Dose									
Grams Carb									
Activity									

Date:	Breakfast	Snack	Lunch	Snack	Dinner	Snack	Bedtime	Night	Notes
Blood Sugar									
Insulin Dose									
Grams Carb									
Activity									

Date:	Breakfast	Snack	Lunch	Snack	Dinner	Snack	Bedtime	Night	Notes
Blood Sugar									
Insulin Dose									
Grams Carb									
Activity									

Date:	Breakfast	Snack	Lunch	Snack	Dinner	Snack	Bedtime	Night	Notes
Blood Sugar									
Insulin Dose									
Grams Carb									
Activity									

Date:	Breakfast	Snack	Lunch	Snack	Dinner	Snack	Bedtime	Night	Notes
Blood Sugar									
Insulin Dose									
Grams Carb									
Activity									

Weekly Diabetes Record

Name: ______________________________

Date:	Breakfast	Snack	Lunch	Snack	Dinner	Snack	Bedtime	Night	Notes
Blood Sugar									
Insulin Dose									
Grams Carb									
Activity									

Date:	Breakfast	Snack	Lunch	Snack	Dinner	Snack	Bedtime	Night	Notes
Blood Sugar									
Insulin Dose									
Grams Carb									
Activity									

Date:	Breakfast	Snack	Lunch	Snack	Dinner	Snack	Bedtime	Night	Notes
Blood Sugar									
Insulin Dose									
Grams Carb									
Activity									

Date:	Breakfast	Snack	Lunch	Snack	Dinner	Snack	Bedtime	Night	Notes
Blood Sugar									
Insulin Dose									
Grams Carb									
Activity									

Date:	Breakfast	Snack	Lunch	Snack	Dinner	Snack	Bedtime	Night	Notes
Blood Sugar									
Insulin Dose									
Grams Carb									
Activity									

Date:	Breakfast	Snack	Lunch	Snack	Dinner	Snack	Bedtime	Night	Notes
Blood Sugar									
Insulin Dose									
Grams Carb									
Activity									

Date:	Breakfast	Snack	Lunch	Snack	Dinner	Snack	Bedtime	Night	Notes
Blood Sugar									
Insulin Dose									
Grams Carb									
Activity									

Weekly Diabetes Record

Name: ______________________________

Date:	Breakfast	Snack	Lunch	Snack	Dinner	Snack	Bedtime	Night	Notes
Blood Sugar									
Insulin Dose									
Grams Carb									
Activity									

Date:	Breakfast	Snack	Lunch	Snack	Dinner	Snack	Bedtime	Night	Notes
Blood Sugar									
Insulin Dose									
Grams Carb									
Activity									

Date:	Breakfast	Snack	Lunch	Snack	Dinner	Snack	Bedtime	Night	Notes
Blood Sugar									
Insulin Dose									
Grams Carb									
Activity									

Date:	Breakfast	Snack	Lunch	Snack	Dinner	Snack	Bedtime	Night	Notes
Blood Sugar									
Insulin Dose									
Grams Carb									
Activity									

Date:	Breakfast	Snack	Lunch	Snack	Dinner	Snack	Bedtime	Night	Notes
Blood Sugar									
Insulin Dose									
Grams Carb									
Activity									

Date:	Breakfast	Snack	Lunch	Snack	Dinner	Snack	Bedtime	Night	Notes
Blood Sugar									
Insulin Dose									
Grams Carb									
Activity									

Date:	Breakfast	Snack	Lunch	Snack	Dinner	Snack	Bedtime	Night	Notes
Blood Sugar									
Insulin Dose									
Grams Carb									
Activity									

Weekly Diabetes Record

Name: ______________________________

Date:	Breakfast	Snack	Lunch	Snack	Dinner	Snack	Bedtime	Night	Notes
Blood Sugar									
Insulin Dose									
Grams Carb									
Activity									

Date:	Breakfast	Snack	Lunch	Snack	Dinner	Snack	Bedtime	Night	Notes
Blood Sugar									
Insulin Dose									
Grams Carb									
Activity									

Date:	Breakfast	Snack	Lunch	Snack	Dinner	Snack	Bedtime	Night	Notes
Blood Sugar									
Insulin Dose									
Grams Carb									
Activity									

Date:	Breakfast	Snack	Lunch	Snack	Dinner	Snack	Bedtime	Night	Notes
Blood Sugar									
Insulin Dose									
Grams Carb									
Activity									

Date:	Breakfast	Snack	Lunch	Snack	Dinner	Snack	Bedtime	Night	Notes
Blood Sugar									
Insulin Dose									
Grams Carb									
Activity									

Date:	Breakfast	Snack	Lunch	Snack	Dinner	Snack	Bedtime	Night	Notes
Blood Sugar									
Insulin Dose									
Grams Carb									
Activity									

Date:	Breakfast	Snack	Lunch	Snack	Dinner	Snack	Bedtime	Night	Notes
Blood Sugar									
Insulin Dose									
Grams Carb									
Activity									

Weekly Diabetes Record

Name: ______________________________

Date:	Breakfast	Snack	Lunch	Snack	Dinner	Snack	Bedtime	Night	Notes
Blood Sugar									
Insulin Dose									
Grams Carb									
Activity									

Date:	Breakfast	Snack	Lunch	Snack	Dinner	Snack	Bedtime	Night	Notes
Blood Sugar									
Insulin Dose									
Grams Carb									
Activity									

Date:	Breakfast	Snack	Lunch	Snack	Dinner	Snack	Bedtime	Night	Notes
Blood Sugar									
Insulin Dose									
Grams Carb									
Activity									

Date:	Breakfast	Snack	Lunch	Snack	Dinner	Snack	Bedtime	Night	Notes
Blood Sugar									
Insulin Dose									
Grams Carb									
Activity									

Date:	Breakfast	Snack	Lunch	Snack	Dinner	Snack	Bedtime	Night	Notes
Blood Sugar									
Insulin Dose									
Grams Carb									
Activity									

Date:	Breakfast	Snack	Lunch	Snack	Dinner	Snack	Bedtime	Night	Notes
Blood Sugar									
Insulin Dose									
Grams Carb									
Activity									

Date:	Breakfast	Snack	Lunch	Snack	Dinner	Snack	Bedtime	Night	Notes
Blood Sugar									
Insulin Dose									
Grams Carb									
Activity									

Weekly Diabetes Record

Name: ______________________________

Date:	Breakfast	Snack	Lunch	Snack	Dinner	Snack	Bedtime	Night	Notes
Blood Sugar									
Insulin Dose									
Grams Carb									
Activity									

Date:	Breakfast	Snack	Lunch	Snack	Dinner	Snack	Bedtime	Night	Notes
Blood Sugar									
Insulin Dose									
Grams Carb									
Activity									

Date:	Breakfast	Snack	Lunch	Snack	Dinner	Snack	Bedtime	Night	Notes
Blood Sugar									
Insulin Dose									
Grams Carb									
Activity									

Date:	Breakfast	Snack	Lunch	Snack	Dinner	Snack	Bedtime	Night	Notes
Blood Sugar									
Insulin Dose									
Grams Carb									
Activity									

Date:	Breakfast	Snack	Lunch	Snack	Dinner	Snack	Bedtime	Night	Notes
Blood Sugar									
Insulin Dose									
Grams Carb									
Activity									

Date:	Breakfast	Snack	Lunch	Snack	Dinner	Snack	Bedtime	Night	Notes
Blood Sugar									
Insulin Dose									
Grams Carb									
Activity									

Date:	Breakfast	Snack	Lunch	Snack	Dinner	Snack	Bedtime	Night	Notes
Blood Sugar									
Insulin Dose									
Grams Carb									
Activity									

Weekly Diabetes Record

Name: ______________________________

Date:	Breakfast	Snack	Lunch	Snack	Dinner	Snack	Bedtime	Night	Notes
Blood Sugar									
Insulin Dose									
Grams Carb									
Activity									

Date:	Breakfast	Snack	Lunch	Snack	Dinner	Snack	Bedtime	Night	Notes
Blood Sugar									
Insulin Dose									
Grams Carb									
Activity									

Date:	Breakfast	Snack	Lunch	Snack	Dinner	Snack	Bedtime	Night	Notes
Blood Sugar									
Insulin Dose									
Grams Carb									
Activity									

Date:	Breakfast	Snack	Lunch	Snack	Dinner	Snack	Bedtime	Night	Notes
Blood Sugar									
Insulin Dose									
Grams Carb									
Activity									

Date:	Breakfast	Snack	Lunch	Snack	Dinner	Snack	Bedtime	Night	Notes
Blood Sugar									
Insulin Dose									
Grams Carb									
Activity									

Date:	Breakfast	Snack	Lunch	Snack	Dinner	Snack	Bedtime	Night	Notes
Blood Sugar									
Insulin Dose									
Grams Carb									
Activity									

Date:	Breakfast	Snack	Lunch	Snack	Dinner	Snack	Bedtime	Night	Notes
Blood Sugar									
Insulin Dose									
Grams Carb									
Activity									

Weekly Diabetes Record

Name: ______________________________

Date:	Breakfast	Snack	Lunch	Snack	Dinner	Snack	Bedtime	Night	Notes
Blood Sugar									
Insulin Dose									
Grams Carb									
Activity									

Date:	Breakfast	Snack	Lunch	Snack	Dinner	Snack	Bedtime	Night	Notes
Blood Sugar									
Insulin Dose									
Grams Carb									
Activity									

Date:	Breakfast	Snack	Lunch	Snack	Dinner	Snack	Bedtime	Night	Notes
Blood Sugar									
Insulin Dose									
Grams Carb									
Activity									

Date:	Breakfast	Snack	Lunch	Snack	Dinner	Snack	Bedtime	Night	Notes
Blood Sugar									
Insulin Dose									
Grams Carb									
Activity									

Date:	Breakfast	Snack	Lunch	Snack	Dinner	Snack	Bedtime	Night	Notes
Blood Sugar									
Insulin Dose									
Grams Carb									
Activity									

Date:	Breakfast	Snack	Lunch	Snack	Dinner	Snack	Bedtime	Night	Notes
Blood Sugar									
Insulin Dose									
Grams Carb									
Activity									

Date:	Breakfast	Snack	Lunch	Snack	Dinner	Snack	Bedtime	Night	Notes
Blood Sugar									
Insulin Dose									
Grams Carb									
Activity									

Weekly Diabetes Record

Name: ______________________________

Date:	Breakfast	Snack	Lunch	Snack	Dinner	Snack	Bedtime	Night	Notes
Blood Sugar									
Insulin Dose									
Grams Carb									
Activity									

Date:	Breakfast	Snack	Lunch	Snack	Dinner	Snack	Bedtime	Night	Notes
Blood Sugar									
Insulin Dose									
Grams Carb									
Activity									

Date:	Breakfast	Snack	Lunch	Snack	Dinner	Snack	Bedtime	Night	Notes
Blood Sugar									
Insulin Dose									
Grams Carb									
Activity									

Date:	Breakfast	Snack	Lunch	Snack	Dinner	Snack	Bedtime	Night	Notes
Blood Sugar									
Insulin Dose									
Grams Carb									
Activity									

Date:	Breakfast	Snack	Lunch	Snack	Dinner	Snack	Bedtime	Night	Notes
Blood Sugar									
Insulin Dose									
Grams Carb									
Activity									

Date:	Breakfast	Snack	Lunch	Snack	Dinner	Snack	Bedtime	Night	Notes
Blood Sugar									
Insulin Dose									
Grams Carb									
Activity									

Date:	Breakfast	Snack	Lunch	Snack	Dinner	Snack	Bedtime	Night	Notes
Blood Sugar									
Insulin Dose									
Grams Carb									
Activity									

Weekly Diabetes Record

Name: ______________________________

Date:	Breakfast	Snack	Lunch	Snack	Dinner	Snack	Bedtime	Night	Notes
Blood Sugar									
Insulin Dose									
Grams Carb									
Activity									

Date:	Breakfast	Snack	Lunch	Snack	Dinner	Snack	Bedtime	Night	Notes
Blood Sugar									
Insulin Dose									
Grams Carb									
Activity									

Date:	Breakfast	Snack	Lunch	Snack	Dinner	Snack	Bedtime	Night	Notes
Blood Sugar									
Insulin Dose									
Grams Carb									
Activity									

Date:	Breakfast	Snack	Lunch	Snack	Dinner	Snack	Bedtime	Night	Notes
Blood Sugar									
Insulin Dose									
Grams Carb									
Activity									

Date:	Breakfast	Snack	Lunch	Snack	Dinner	Snack	Bedtime	Night	Notes
Blood Sugar									
Insulin Dose									
Grams Carb									
Activity									

Date:	Breakfast	Snack	Lunch	Snack	Dinner	Snack	Bedtime	Night	Notes
Blood Sugar									
Insulin Dose									
Grams Carb									
Activity									

Date:	Breakfast	Snack	Lunch	Snack	Dinner	Snack	Bedtime	Night	Notes
Blood Sugar									
Insulin Dose									
Grams Carb									
Activity									

Weekly Diabetes Record

Name: ____

Date:	Breakfast	Snack	Lunch	Snack	Dinner	Snack	Bedtime	Night	Notes
Blood Sugar									
Insulin Dose									
Grams Carb									
Activity									

Date:	Breakfast	Snack	Lunch	Snack	Dinner	Snack	Bedtime	Night	Notes
Blood Sugar									
Insulin Dose									
Grams Carb									
Activity									

Date:	Breakfast	Snack	Lunch	Snack	Dinner	Snack	Bedtime	Night	Notes
Blood Sugar									
Insulin Dose									
Grams Carb									
Activity									

Date:	Breakfast	Snack	Lunch	Snack	Dinner	Snack	Bedtime	Night	Notes
Blood Sugar									
Insulin Dose									
Grams Carb									
Activity									

Date:	Breakfast	Snack	Lunch	Snack	Dinner	Snack	Bedtime	Night	Notes
Blood Sugar									
Insulin Dose									
Grams Carb									
Activity									

Date:	Breakfast	Snack	Lunch	Snack	Dinner	Snack	Bedtime	Night	Notes
Blood Sugar									
Insulin Dose									
Grams Carb									
Activity									

Date:	Breakfast	Snack	Lunch	Snack	Dinner	Snack	Bedtime	Night	Notes
Blood Sugar									
Insulin Dose									
Grams Carb									
Activity									

Weekly Diabetes Record

Name: ______________________________

Date:	Breakfast	Snack	Lunch	Snack	Dinner	Snack	Bedtime	Night	Notes
Blood Sugar									
Insulin Dose									
Grams Carb									
Activity									

Date:	Breakfast	Snack	Lunch	Snack	Dinner	Snack	Bedtime	Night	Notes
Blood Sugar									
Insulin Dose									
Grams Carb									
Activity									

Date:	Breakfast	Snack	Lunch	Snack	Dinner	Snack	Bedtime	Night	Notes
Blood Sugar									
Insulin Dose									
Grams Carb									
Activity									

Date:	Breakfast	Snack	Lunch	Snack	Dinner	Snack	Bedtime	Night	Notes
Blood Sugar									
Insulin Dose									
Grams Carb									
Activity									

Date:	Breakfast	Snack	Lunch	Snack	Dinner	Snack	Bedtime	Night	Notes
Blood Sugar									
Insulin Dose									
Grams Carb									
Activity									

Date:	Breakfast	Snack	Lunch	Snack	Dinner	Snack	Bedtime	Night	Notes
Blood Sugar									
Insulin Dose									
Grams Carb									
Activity									

Date:	Breakfast	Snack	Lunch	Snack	Dinner	Snack	Bedtime	Night	Notes
Blood Sugar									
Insulin Dose									
Grams Carb									
Activity									

Weekly Diabetes Record

Name: ______________________________

Date:	Breakfast	Snack	Lunch	Snack	Dinner	Snack	Bedtime	Night	Notes
Blood Sugar									
Insulin Dose									
Grams Carb									
Activity									

Date:	Breakfast	Snack	Lunch	Snack	Dinner	Snack	Bedtime	Night	Notes
Blood Sugar									
Insulin Dose									
Grams Carb									
Activity									

Date:	Breakfast	Snack	Lunch	Snack	Dinner	Snack	Bedtime	Night	Notes
Blood Sugar									
Insulin Dose									
Grams Carb									
Activity									

Date:	Breakfast	Snack	Lunch	Snack	Dinner	Snack	Bedtime	Night	Notes
Blood Sugar									
Insulin Dose									
Grams Carb									
Activity									

Date:	Breakfast	Snack	Lunch	Snack	Dinner	Snack	Bedtime	Night	Notes
Blood Sugar									
Insulin Dose									
Grams Carb									
Activity									

Date:	Breakfast	Snack	Lunch	Snack	Dinner	Snack	Bedtime	Night	Notes
Blood Sugar									
Insulin Dose									
Grams Carb									
Activity									

Date:	Breakfast	Snack	Lunch	Snack	Dinner	Snack	Bedtime	Night	Notes
Blood Sugar									
Insulin Dose									
Grams Carb									
Activity									

Weekly Diabetes Record

Name: ______________________________

Date:	Breakfast	Snack	Lunch	Snack	Dinner	Snack	Bedtime	Night	Notes
Blood Sugar									
Insulin Dose									
Grams Carb									
Activity									

Date:	Breakfast	Snack	Lunch	Snack	Dinner	Snack	Bedtime	Night	Notes
Blood Sugar									
Insulin Dose									
Grams Carb									
Activity									

Date:	Breakfast	Snack	Lunch	Snack	Dinner	Snack	Bedtime	Night	Notes
Blood Sugar									
Insulin Dose									
Grams Carb									
Activity									

Date:	Breakfast	Snack	Lunch	Snack	Dinner	Snack	Bedtime	Night	Notes
Blood Sugar									
Insulin Dose									
Grams Carb									
Activity									

Date:	Breakfast	Snack	Lunch	Snack	Dinner	Snack	Bedtime	Night	Notes
Blood Sugar									
Insulin Dose									
Grams Carb									
Activity									

Date:	Breakfast	Snack	Lunch	Snack	Dinner	Snack	Bedtime	Night	Notes
Blood Sugar									
Insulin Dose									
Grams Carb									
Activity									

Date:	Breakfast	Snack	Lunch	Snack	Dinner	Snack	Bedtime	Night	Notes
Blood Sugar									
Insulin Dose									
Grams Carb									
Activity									

Weekly Diabetes Record

Name: ____________________

Date:	Breakfast	Snack	Lunch	Snack	Dinner	Snack	Bedtime	Night	Notes
Blood Sugar									
Insulin Dose									
Grams Carb									
Activity									

Date:	Breakfast	Snack	Lunch	Snack	Dinner	Snack	Bedtime	Night	Notes
Blood Sugar									
Insulin Dose									
Grams Carb									
Activity									

Date:	Breakfast	Snack	Lunch	Snack	Dinner	Snack	Bedtime	Night	Notes
Blood Sugar									
Insulin Dose									
Grams Carb									
Activity									

Date:	Breakfast	Snack	Lunch	Snack	Dinner	Snack	Bedtime	Night	Notes
Blood Sugar									
Insulin Dose									
Grams Carb									
Activity									

Date:	Breakfast	Snack	Lunch	Snack	Dinner	Snack	Bedtime	Night	Notes
Blood Sugar									
Insulin Dose									
Grams Carb									
Activity									

Date:	Breakfast	Snack	Lunch	Snack	Dinner	Snack	Bedtime	Night	Notes
Blood Sugar									
Insulin Dose									
Grams Carb									
Activity									

Date:	Breakfast	Snack	Lunch	Snack	Dinner	Snack	Bedtime	Night	Notes
Blood Sugar									
Insulin Dose									
Grams Carb									
Activity									

Weekly Diabetes Record

Name: ______________________________

Date:	Breakfast	Snack	Lunch	Snack	Dinner	Snack	Bedtime	Night	Notes
Blood Sugar									
Insulin Dose									
Grams Carb									
Activity									

Date:	Breakfast	Snack	Lunch	Snack	Dinner	Snack	Bedtime	Night	Notes
Blood Sugar									
Insulin Dose									
Grams Carb									
Activity									

Date:	Breakfast	Snack	Lunch	Snack	Dinner	Snack	Bedtime	Night	Notes
Blood Sugar									
Insulin Dose									
Grams Carb									
Activity									

Date:	Breakfast	Snack	Lunch	Snack	Dinner	Snack	Bedtime	Night	Notes
Blood Sugar									
Insulin Dose									
Grams Carb									
Activity									

Date:	Breakfast	Snack	Lunch	Snack	Dinner	Snack	Bedtime	Night	Notes
Blood Sugar									
Insulin Dose									
Grams Carb									
Activity									

Date:	Breakfast	Snack	Lunch	Snack	Dinner	Snack	Bedtime	Night	Notes
Blood Sugar									
Insulin Dose									
Grams Carb									
Activity									

Date:	Breakfast	Snack	Lunch	Snack	Dinner	Snack	Bedtime	Night	Notes
Blood Sugar									
Insulin Dose									
Grams Carb									
Activity									

Weekly Diabetes Record

Name: ______________________________________

Date:	Breakfast	Snack	Lunch	Snack	Dinner	Snack	Bedtime	Night	Notes
Blood Sugar									
Insulin Dose									
Grams Carb									
Activity									

Date:	Breakfast	Snack	Lunch	Snack	Dinner	Snack	Bedtime	Night	Notes
Blood Sugar									
Insulin Dose									
Grams Carb									
Activity									

Date:	Breakfast	Snack	Lunch	Snack	Dinner	Snack	Bedtime	Night	Notes
Blood Sugar									
Insulin Dose									
Grams Carb									
Activity									

Date:	Breakfast	Snack	Lunch	Snack	Dinner	Snack	Bedtime	Night	Notes
Blood Sugar									
Insulin Dose									
Grams Carb									
Activity									

Date:	Breakfast	Snack	Lunch	Snack	Dinner	Snack	Bedtime	Night	Notes
Blood Sugar									
Insulin Dose									
Grams Carb									
Activity									

Date:	Breakfast	Snack	Lunch	Snack	Dinner	Snack	Bedtime	Night	Notes
Blood Sugar									
Insulin Dose									
Grams Carb									
Activity									

Date:	Breakfast	Snack	Lunch	Snack	Dinner	Snack	Bedtime	Night	Notes
Blood Sugar									
Insulin Dose									
Grams Carb									
Activity									

Weekly Diabetes Record

Name: ______________________________

Date:	Breakfast	Snack	Lunch	Snack	Dinner	Snack	Bedtime	Night	Notes
Blood Sugar									
Insulin Dose									
Grams Carb									
Activity									

Date:	Breakfast	Snack	Lunch	Snack	Dinner	Snack	Bedtime	Night	Notes
Blood Sugar									
Insulin Dose									
Grams Carb									
Activity									

Date:	Breakfast	Snack	Lunch	Snack	Dinner	Snack	Bedtime	Night	Notes
Blood Sugar									
Insulin Dose									
Grams Carb									
Activity									

Date:	Breakfast	Snack	Lunch	Snack	Dinner	Snack	Bedtime	Night	Notes
Blood Sugar									
Insulin Dose									
Grams Carb									
Activity									

Date:	Breakfast	Snack	Lunch	Snack	Dinner	Snack	Bedtime	Night	Notes
Blood Sugar									
Insulin Dose									
Grams Carb									
Activity									

Date:	Breakfast	Snack	Lunch	Snack	Dinner	Snack	Bedtime	Night	Notes
Blood Sugar									
Insulin Dose									
Grams Carb									
Activity									

Date:	Breakfast	Snack	Lunch	Snack	Dinner	Snack	Bedtime	Night	Notes
Blood Sugar									
Insulin Dose									
Grams Carb									
Activity									

Weekly Diabetes Record

Name: ____

Date:	Breakfast	Snack	Lunch	Snack	Dinner	Snack	Bedtime	Night	Notes
Blood Sugar									
Insulin Dose									
Grams Carb									
Activity									

Date:	Breakfast	Snack	Lunch	Snack	Dinner	Snack	Bedtime	Night	Notes
Blood Sugar									
Insulin Dose									
Grams Carb									
Activity									

Date:	Breakfast	Snack	Lunch	Snack	Dinner	Snack	Bedtime	Night	Notes
Blood Sugar									
Insulin Dose									
Grams Carb									
Activity									

Date:	Breakfast	Snack	Lunch	Snack	Dinner	Snack	Bedtime	Night	Notes
Blood Sugar									
Insulin Dose									
Grams Carb									
Activity									

Date:	Breakfast	Snack	Lunch	Snack	Dinner	Snack	Bedtime	Night	Notes
Blood Sugar									
Insulin Dose									
Grams Carb									
Activity									

Date:	Breakfast	Snack	Lunch	Snack	Dinner	Snack	Bedtime	Night	Notes
Blood Sugar									
Insulin Dose									
Grams Carb									
Activity									

Date:	Breakfast	Snack	Lunch	Snack	Dinner	Snack	Bedtime	Night	Notes
Blood Sugar									
Insulin Dose									
Grams Carb									
Activity									

Weekly Diabetes Record

Name: ____

Date:	Breakfast	Snack	Lunch	Snack	Dinner	Snack	Bedtime	Night	Notes
Blood Sugar									
Insulin Dose									
Grams Carb									
Activity									

Date:	Breakfast	Snack	Lunch	Snack	Dinner	Snack	Bedtime	Night	Notes
Blood Sugar									
Insulin Dose									
Grams Carb									
Activity									

Date:	Breakfast	Snack	Lunch	Snack	Dinner	Snack	Bedtime	Night	Notes
Blood Sugar									
Insulin Dose									
Grams Carb									
Activity									

Date:	Breakfast	Snack	Lunch	Snack	Dinner	Snack	Bedtime	Night	Notes
Blood Sugar									
Insulin Dose									
Grams Carb									
Activity									

Date:	Breakfast	Snack	Lunch	Snack	Dinner	Snack	Bedtime	Night	Notes
Blood Sugar									
Insulin Dose									
Grams Carb									
Activity									

Date:	Breakfast	Snack	Lunch	Snack	Dinner	Snack	Bedtime	Night	Notes
Blood Sugar									
Insulin Dose									
Grams Carb									
Activity									

Date:	Breakfast	Snack	Lunch	Snack	Dinner	Snack	Bedtime	Night	Notes
Blood Sugar									
Insulin Dose									
Grams Carb									
Activity									

Weekly Diabetes Record

Name: ______________________________

Date:	Breakfast	Snack	Lunch	Snack	Dinner	Snack	Bedtime	Night	Notes
Blood Sugar									
Insulin Dose									
Grams Carb									
Activity									

Date:	Breakfast	Snack	Lunch	Snack	Dinner	Snack	Bedtime	Night	Notes
Blood Sugar									
Insulin Dose									
Grams Carb									
Activity									

Date:	Breakfast	Snack	Lunch	Snack	Dinner	Snack	Bedtime	Night	Notes
Blood Sugar									
Insulin Dose									
Grams Carb									
Activity									

Date:	Breakfast	Snack	Lunch	Snack	Dinner	Snack	Bedtime	Night	Notes
Blood Sugar									
Insulin Dose									
Grams Carb									
Activity									

Date:	Breakfast	Snack	Lunch	Snack	Dinner	Snack	Bedtime	Night	Notes
Blood Sugar									
Insulin Dose									
Grams Carb									
Activity									

Date:	Breakfast	Snack	Lunch	Snack	Dinner	Snack	Bedtime	Night	Notes
Blood Sugar									
Insulin Dose									
Grams Carb									
Activity									

Date:	Breakfast	Snack	Lunch	Snack	Dinner	Snack	Bedtime	Night	Notes
Blood Sugar									
Insulin Dose									
Grams Carb									
Activity									

Weekly Diabetes Record

Name: ________________________________

Date:	Breakfast	Snack	Lunch	Snack	Dinner	Snack	Bedtime	Night	Notes
Blood Sugar									
Insulin Dose									
Grams Carb									
Activity									

Date:	Breakfast	Snack	Lunch	Snack	Dinner	Snack	Bedtime	Night	Notes
Blood Sugar									
Insulin Dose									
Grams Carb									
Activity									

Date:	Breakfast	Snack	Lunch	Snack	Dinner	Snack	Bedtime	Night	Notes
Blood Sugar									
Insulin Dose									
Grams Carb									
Activity									

Date:	Breakfast	Snack	Lunch	Snack	Dinner	Snack	Bedtime	Night	Notes
Blood Sugar									
Insulin Dose									
Grams Carb									
Activity									

Date:	Breakfast	Snack	Lunch	Snack	Dinner	Snack	Bedtime	Night	Notes
Blood Sugar									
Insulin Dose									
Grams Carb									
Activity									

Date:	Breakfast	Snack	Lunch	Snack	Dinner	Snack	Bedtime	Night	Notes
Blood Sugar									
Insulin Dose									
Grams Carb									
Activity									

Date:	Breakfast	Snack	Lunch	Snack	Dinner	Snack	Bedtime	Night	Notes
Blood Sugar									
Insulin Dose									
Grams Carb									
Activity									

Weekly Diabetes Record

Name: ______________________________

Date:	Breakfast	Snack	Lunch	Snack	Dinner	Snack	Bedtime	Night	Notes
Blood Sugar									
Insulin Dose									
Grams Carb									
Activity									

Date:	Breakfast	Snack	Lunch	Snack	Dinner	Snack	Bedtime	Night	Notes
Blood Sugar									
Insulin Dose									
Grams Carb									
Activity									

Date:	Breakfast	Snack	Lunch	Snack	Dinner	Snack	Bedtime	Night	Notes
Blood Sugar									
Insulin Dose									
Grams Carb									
Activity									

Date:	Breakfast	Snack	Lunch	Snack	Dinner	Snack	Bedtime	Night	Notes
Blood Sugar									
Insulin Dose									
Grams Carb									
Activity									

Date:	Breakfast	Snack	Lunch	Snack	Dinner	Snack	Bedtime	Night	Notes
Blood Sugar									
Insulin Dose									
Grams Carb									
Activity									

Date:	Breakfast	Snack	Lunch	Snack	Dinner	Snack	Bedtime	Night	Notes
Blood Sugar									
Insulin Dose									
Grams Carb									
Activity									

Date:	Breakfast	Snack	Lunch	Snack	Dinner	Snack	Bedtime	Night	Notes
Blood Sugar									
Insulin Dose									
Grams Carb									
Activity									

Weekly Diabetes Record

Name: ______________________________

Date:	Breakfast	Snack	Lunch	Snack	Dinner	Snack	Bedtime	Night	Notes
Blood Sugar									
Insulin Dose									
Grams Carb									
Activity									

Date:	Breakfast	Snack	Lunch	Snack	Dinner	Snack	Bedtime	Night	Notes
Blood Sugar									
Insulin Dose									
Grams Carb									
Activity									

Date:	Breakfast	Snack	Lunch	Snack	Dinner	Snack	Bedtime	Night	Notes
Blood Sugar									
Insulin Dose									
Grams Carb									
Activity									

Date:	Breakfast	Snack	Lunch	Snack	Dinner	Snack	Bedtime	Night	Notes
Blood Sugar									
Insulin Dose									
Grams Carb									
Activity									

Date:	Breakfast	Snack	Lunch	Snack	Dinner	Snack	Bedtime	Night	Notes
Blood Sugar									
Insulin Dose									
Grams Carb									
Activity									

Date:	Breakfast	Snack	Lunch	Snack	Dinner	Snack	Bedtime	Night	Notes
Blood Sugar									
Insulin Dose									
Grams Carb									
Activity									

Date:	Breakfast	Snack	Lunch	Snack	Dinner	Snack	Bedtime	Night	Notes
Blood Sugar									
Insulin Dose									
Grams Carb									
Activity									

Weekly Diabetes Record

Name: ______________________________

Date:	Breakfast	Snack	Lunch	Snack	Dinner	Snack	Bedtime	Night	Notes
Blood Sugar									
Insulin Dose									
Grams Carb									
Activity									

Date:	Breakfast	Snack	Lunch	Snack	Dinner	Snack	Bedtime	Night	Notes
Blood Sugar									
Insulin Dose									
Grams Carb									
Activity									

Date:	Breakfast	Snack	Lunch	Snack	Dinner	Snack	Bedtime	Night	Notes
Blood Sugar									
Insulin Dose									
Grams Carb									
Activity									

Date:	Breakfast	Snack	Lunch	Snack	Dinner	Snack	Bedtime	Night	Notes
Blood Sugar									
Insulin Dose									
Grams Carb									
Activity									

Date:	Breakfast	Snack	Lunch	Snack	Dinner	Snack	Bedtime	Night	Notes
Blood Sugar									
Insulin Dose									
Grams Carb									
Activity									

Date:	Breakfast	Snack	Lunch	Snack	Dinner	Snack	Bedtime	Night	Notes
Blood Sugar									
Insulin Dose									
Grams Carb									
Activity									

Date:	Breakfast	Snack	Lunch	Snack	Dinner	Snack	Bedtime	Night	Notes
Blood Sugar									
Insulin Dose									
Grams Carb									
Activity									

Weekly Diabetes Record

Name: ____________________________

Date:	Breakfast	Snack	Lunch	Snack	Dinner	Snack	Bedtime	Night	Notes
Blood Sugar									
Insulin Dose									
Grams Carb									
Activity									

Date:	Breakfast	Snack	Lunch	Snack	Dinner	Snack	Bedtime	Night	Notes
Blood Sugar									
Insulin Dose									
Grams Carb									
Activity									

Date:	Breakfast	Snack	Lunch	Snack	Dinner	Snack	Bedtime	Night	Notes
Blood Sugar									
Insulin Dose									
Grams Carb									
Activity									

Date:	Breakfast	Snack	Lunch	Snack	Dinner	Snack	Bedtime	Night	Notes
Blood Sugar									
Insulin Dose									
Grams Carb									
Activity									

Date:	Breakfast	Snack	Lunch	Snack	Dinner	Snack	Bedtime	Night	Notes
Blood Sugar									
Insulin Dose									
Grams Carb									
Activity									

Date:	Breakfast	Snack	Lunch	Snack	Dinner	Snack	Bedtime	Night	Notes
Blood Sugar									
Insulin Dose									
Grams Carb									
Activity									

Date:	Breakfast	Snack	Lunch	Snack	Dinner	Snack	Bedtime	Night	Notes
Blood Sugar									
Insulin Dose									
Grams Carb									
Activity									

Weekly Diabetes Record

Name: ____

Date:	Breakfast	Snack	Lunch	Snack	Dinner	Snack	Bedtime	Night	Notes
Blood Sugar									
Insulin Dose									
Grams Carb									
Activity									

Date:	Breakfast	Snack	Lunch	Snack	Dinner	Snack	Bedtime	Night	Notes
Blood Sugar									
Insulin Dose									
Grams Carb									
Activity									

Date:	Breakfast	Snack	Lunch	Snack	Dinner	Snack	Bedtime	Night	Notes
Blood Sugar									
Insulin Dose									
Grams Carb									
Activity									

Date:	Breakfast	Snack	Lunch	Snack	Dinner	Snack	Bedtime	Night	Notes
Blood Sugar									
Insulin Dose									
Grams Carb									
Activity									

Date:	Breakfast	Snack	Lunch	Snack	Dinner	Snack	Bedtime	Night	Notes
Blood Sugar									
Insulin Dose									
Grams Carb									
Activity									

Date:	Breakfast	Snack	Lunch	Snack	Dinner	Snack	Bedtime	Night	Notes
Blood Sugar									
Insulin Dose									
Grams Carb									
Activity									

Date:	Breakfast	Snack	Lunch	Snack	Dinner	Snack	Bedtime	Night	Notes
Blood Sugar									
Insulin Dose									
Grams Carb									
Activity									

Weekly Diabetes Record

Name: ______________________________

Date:	Breakfast	Snack	Lunch	Snack	Dinner	Snack	Bedtime	Night	Notes
Blood Sugar									
Insulin Dose									
Grams Carb									
Activity									

Date:	Breakfast	Snack	Lunch	Snack	Dinner	Snack	Bedtime	Night	Notes
Blood Sugar									
Insulin Dose									
Grams Carb									
Activity									

Date:	Breakfast	Snack	Lunch	Snack	Dinner	Snack	Bedtime	Night	Notes
Blood Sugar									
Insulin Dose									
Grams Carb									
Activity									

Date:	Breakfast	Snack	Lunch	Snack	Dinner	Snack	Bedtime	Night	Notes
Blood Sugar									
Insulin Dose									
Grams Carb									
Activity									

Date:	Breakfast	Snack	Lunch	Snack	Dinner	Snack	Bedtime	Night	Notes
Blood Sugar									
Insulin Dose									
Grams Carb									
Activity									

Date:	Breakfast	Snack	Lunch	Snack	Dinner	Snack	Bedtime	Night	Notes
Blood Sugar									
Insulin Dose									
Grams Carb									
Activity									

Date:	Breakfast	Snack	Lunch	Snack	Dinner	Snack	Bedtime	Night	Notes
Blood Sugar									
Insulin Dose									
Grams Carb									
Activity									

Weekly Diabetes Record

Name: ______________________________

Date:	Breakfast	Snack	Lunch	Snack	Dinner	Snack	Bedtime	Night	Notes
Blood Sugar									
Insulin Dose									
Grams Carb									
Activity									

Date:	Breakfast	Snack	Lunch	Snack	Dinner	Snack	Bedtime	Night	Notes
Blood Sugar									
Insulin Dose									
Grams Carb									
Activity									

Date:	Breakfast	Snack	Lunch	Snack	Dinner	Snack	Bedtime	Night	Notes
Blood Sugar									
Insulin Dose									
Grams Carb									
Activity									

Date:	Breakfast	Snack	Lunch	Snack	Dinner	Snack	Bedtime	Night	Notes
Blood Sugar									
Insulin Dose									
Grams Carb									
Activity									

Date:	Breakfast	Snack	Lunch	Snack	Dinner	Snack	Bedtime	Night	Notes
Blood Sugar									
Insulin Dose									
Grams Carb									
Activity									

Date:	Breakfast	Snack	Lunch	Snack	Dinner	Snack	Bedtime	Night	Notes
Blood Sugar									
Insulin Dose									
Grams Carb									
Activity									

Date:	Breakfast	Snack	Lunch	Snack	Dinner	Snack	Bedtime	Night	Notes
Blood Sugar									
Insulin Dose									
Grams Carb									
Activity									

Weekly Diabetes Record

Name: ______________________________

Date:	Breakfast	Snack	Lunch	Snack	Dinner	Snack	Bedtime	Night	Notes
Blood Sugar									
Insulin Dose									
Grams Carb									
Activity									

Date:	Breakfast	Snack	Lunch	Snack	Dinner	Snack	Bedtime	Night	Notes
Blood Sugar									
Insulin Dose									
Grams Carb									
Activity									

Date:	Breakfast	Snack	Lunch	Snack	Dinner	Snack	Bedtime	Night	Notes
Blood Sugar									
Insulin Dose									
Grams Carb									
Activity									

Date:	Breakfast	Snack	Lunch	Snack	Dinner	Snack	Bedtime	Night	Notes
Blood Sugar									
Insulin Dose									
Grams Carb									
Activity									

Date:	Breakfast	Snack	Lunch	Snack	Dinner	Snack	Bedtime	Night	Notes
Blood Sugar									
Insulin Dose									
Grams Carb									
Activity									

Date:	Breakfast	Snack	Lunch	Snack	Dinner	Snack	Bedtime	Night	Notes
Blood Sugar									
Insulin Dose									
Grams Carb									
Activity									

Date:	Breakfast	Snack	Lunch	Snack	Dinner	Snack	Bedtime	Night	Notes
Blood Sugar									
Insulin Dose									
Grams Carb									
Activity									

Weekly Diabetes Record

Name: ___________________________________

Date:	Breakfast	Snack	Lunch	Snack	Dinner	Snack	Bedtime	Night	Notes
Blood Sugar									
Insulin Dose									
Grams Carb									
Activity									

Date:	Breakfast	Snack	Lunch	Snack	Dinner	Snack	Bedtime	Night	Notes
Blood Sugar									
Insulin Dose									
Grams Carb									
Activity									

Date:	Breakfast	Snack	Lunch	Snack	Dinner	Snack	Bedtime	Night	Notes
Blood Sugar									
Insulin Dose									
Grams Carb									
Activity									

Date:	Breakfast	Snack	Lunch	Snack	Dinner	Snack	Bedtime	Night	Notes
Blood Sugar									
Insulin Dose									
Grams Carb									
Activity									

Date:	Breakfast	Snack	Lunch	Snack	Dinner	Snack	Bedtime	Night	Notes
Blood Sugar									
Insulin Dose									
Grams Carb									
Activity									

Date:	Breakfast	Snack	Lunch	Snack	Dinner	Snack	Bedtime	Night	Notes
Blood Sugar									
Insulin Dose									
Grams Carb									
Activity									

Date:	Breakfast	Snack	Lunch	Snack	Dinner	Snack	Bedtime	Night	Notes
Blood Sugar									
Insulin Dose									
Grams Carb									
Activity									

Weekly Diabetes Record

Name: ______________________________

Date:	Breakfast	Snack	Lunch	Snack	Dinner	Snack	Bedtime	Night	Notes
Blood Sugar									
Insulin Dose									
Grams Carb									
Activity									

Date:	Breakfast	Snack	Lunch	Snack	Dinner	Snack	Bedtime	Night	Notes
Blood Sugar									
Insulin Dose									
Grams Carb									
Activity									

Date:	Breakfast	Snack	Lunch	Snack	Dinner	Snack	Bedtime	Night	Notes
Blood Sugar									
Insulin Dose									
Grams Carb									
Activity									

Date:	Breakfast	Snack	Lunch	Snack	Dinner	Snack	Bedtime	Night	Notes
Blood Sugar									
Insulin Dose									
Grams Carb									
Activity									

Date:	Breakfast	Snack	Lunch	Snack	Dinner	Snack	Bedtime	Night	Notes
Blood Sugar									
Insulin Dose									
Grams Carb									
Activity									

Date:	Breakfast	Snack	Lunch	Snack	Dinner	Snack	Bedtime	Night	Notes
Blood Sugar									
Insulin Dose									
Grams Carb									
Activity									

Date:	Breakfast	Snack	Lunch	Snack	Dinner	Snack	Bedtime	Night	Notes
Blood Sugar									
Insulin Dose									
Grams Carb									
Activity									

Weekly Diabetes Record

Name: ____________________

Date:	Breakfast	Snack	Lunch	Snack	Dinner	Snack	Bedtime	Night	Notes
Blood Sugar									
Insulin Dose									
Grams Carb									
Activity									

Date:	Breakfast	Snack	Lunch	Snack	Dinner	Snack	Bedtime	Night	Notes
Blood Sugar									
Insulin Dose									
Grams Carb									
Activity									

Date:	Breakfast	Snack	Lunch	Snack	Dinner	Snack	Bedtime	Night	Notes
Blood Sugar									
Insulin Dose									
Grams Carb									
Activity									

Date:	Breakfast	Snack	Lunch	Snack	Dinner	Snack	Bedtime	Night	Notes
Blood Sugar									
Insulin Dose									
Grams Carb									
Activity									

Date:	Breakfast	Snack	Lunch	Snack	Dinner	Snack	Bedtime	Night	Notes
Blood Sugar									
Insulin Dose									
Grams Carb									
Activity									

Date:	Breakfast	Snack	Lunch	Snack	Dinner	Snack	Bedtime	Night	Notes
Blood Sugar									
Insulin Dose									
Grams Carb									
Activity									

Date:	Breakfast	Snack	Lunch	Snack	Dinner	Snack	Bedtime	Night	Notes
Blood Sugar									
Insulin Dose									
Grams Carb									
Activity									

Weekly Diabetes Record

Name: ______________________________

Date:	Breakfast	Snack	Lunch	Snack	Dinner	Snack	Bedtime	Night	Notes
Blood Sugar									
Insulin Dose									
Grams Carb									
Activity									

Date:	Breakfast	Snack	Lunch	Snack	Dinner	Snack	Bedtime	Night	Notes
Blood Sugar									
Insulin Dose									
Grams Carb									
Activity									

Date:	Breakfast	Snack	Lunch	Snack	Dinner	Snack	Bedtime	Night	Notes
Blood Sugar									
Insulin Dose									
Grams Carb									
Activity									

Date:	Breakfast	Snack	Lunch	Snack	Dinner	Snack	Bedtime	Night	Notes
Blood Sugar									
Insulin Dose									
Grams Carb									
Activity									

Date:	Breakfast	Snack	Lunch	Snack	Dinner	Snack	Bedtime	Night	Notes
Blood Sugar									
Insulin Dose									
Grams Carb									
Activity									

Date:	Breakfast	Snack	Lunch	Snack	Dinner	Snack	Bedtime	Night	Notes
Blood Sugar									
Insulin Dose									
Grams Carb									
Activity									

Date:	Breakfast	Snack	Lunch	Snack	Dinner	Snack	Bedtime	Night	Notes
Blood Sugar									
Insulin Dose									
Grams Carb									
Activity									

Weekly Diabetes Record

Name: ____________________________________

Date:	Breakfast	Snack	Lunch	Snack	Dinner	Snack	Bedtime	Night	Notes
Blood Sugar									
Insulin Dose									
Grams Carb									
Activity									

Date:	Breakfast	Snack	Lunch	Snack	Dinner	Snack	Bedtime	Night	Notes
Blood Sugar									
Insulin Dose									
Grams Carb									
Activity									

Date:	Breakfast	Snack	Lunch	Snack	Dinner	Snack	Bedtime	Night	Notes
Blood Sugar									
Insulin Dose									
Grams Carb									
Activity									

Date:	Breakfast	Snack	Lunch	Snack	Dinner	Snack	Bedtime	Night	Notes
Blood Sugar									
Insulin Dose									
Grams Carb									
Activity									

Date:	Breakfast	Snack	Lunch	Snack	Dinner	Snack	Bedtime	Night	Notes
Blood Sugar									
Insulin Dose									
Grams Carb									
Activity									

Date:	Breakfast	Snack	Lunch	Snack	Dinner	Snack	Bedtime	Night	Notes
Blood Sugar									
Insulin Dose									
Grams Carb									
Activity									

Date:	Breakfast	Snack	Lunch	Snack	Dinner	Snack	Bedtime	Night	Notes
Blood Sugar									
Insulin Dose									
Grams Carb									
Activity									

Weekly Diabetes Record

Name: ____________________

Date:	Breakfast	Snack	Lunch	Snack	Dinner	Snack	Bedtime	Night	Notes
Blood Sugar									
Insulin Dose									
Grams Carb									
Activity									

Date:	Breakfast	Snack	Lunch	Snack	Dinner	Snack	Bedtime	Night	Notes
Blood Sugar									
Insulin Dose									
Grams Carb									
Activity									

Date:	Breakfast	Snack	Lunch	Snack	Dinner	Snack	Bedtime	Night	Notes
Blood Sugar									
Insulin Dose									
Grams Carb									
Activity									

Date:	Breakfast	Snack	Lunch	Snack	Dinner	Snack	Bedtime	Night	Notes
Blood Sugar									
Insulin Dose									
Grams Carb									
Activity									

Date:	Breakfast	Snack	Lunch	Snack	Dinner	Snack	Bedtime	Night	Notes
Blood Sugar									
Insulin Dose									
Grams Carb									
Activity									

Date:	Breakfast	Snack	Lunch	Snack	Dinner	Snack	Bedtime	Night	Notes
Blood Sugar									
Insulin Dose									
Grams Carb									
Activity									

Date:	Breakfast	Snack	Lunch	Snack	Dinner	Snack	Bedtime	Night	Notes
Blood Sugar									
Insulin Dose									
Grams Carb									
Activity									

Weekly Diabetes Record

Name: ______________________________

Date:	Breakfast	Snack	Lunch	Snack	Dinner	Snack	Bedtime	Night	Notes
Blood Sugar									
Insulin Dose									
Grams Carb									
Activity									

Date:	Breakfast	Snack	Lunch	Snack	Dinner	Snack	Bedtime	Night	Notes
Blood Sugar									
Insulin Dose									
Grams Carb									
Activity									

Date:	Breakfast	Snack	Lunch	Snack	Dinner	Snack	Bedtime	Night	Notes
Blood Sugar									
Insulin Dose									
Grams Carb									
Activity									

Date:	Breakfast	Snack	Lunch	Snack	Dinner	Snack	Bedtime	Night	Notes
Blood Sugar									
Insulin Dose									
Grams Carb									
Activity									

Date:	Breakfast	Snack	Lunch	Snack	Dinner	Snack	Bedtime	Night	Notes
Blood Sugar									
Insulin Dose									
Grams Carb									
Activity									

Date:	Breakfast	Snack	Lunch	Snack	Dinner	Snack	Bedtime	Night	Notes
Blood Sugar									
Insulin Dose									
Grams Carb									
Activity									

Date:	Breakfast	Snack	Lunch	Snack	Dinner	Snack	Bedtime	Night	Notes
Blood Sugar									
Insulin Dose									
Grams Carb									
Activity									

Weekly Diabetes Record

Name: ______________________________

Date:	Breakfast	Snack	Lunch	Snack	Dinner	Snack	Bedtime	Night	Notes
Blood Sugar									
Insulin Dose									
Grams Carb									
Activity									

Date:	Breakfast	Snack	Lunch	Snack	Dinner	Snack	Bedtime	Night	Notes
Blood Sugar									
Insulin Dose									
Grams Carb									
Activity									

Date:	Breakfast	Snack	Lunch	Snack	Dinner	Snack	Bedtime	Night	Notes
Blood Sugar									
Insulin Dose									
Grams Carb									
Activity									

Date:	Breakfast	Snack	Lunch	Snack	Dinner	Snack	Bedtime	Night	Notes
Blood Sugar									
Insulin Dose									
Grams Carb									
Activity									

Date:	Breakfast	Snack	Lunch	Snack	Dinner	Snack	Bedtime	Night	Notes
Blood Sugar									
Insulin Dose									
Grams Carb									
Activity									

Date:	Breakfast	Snack	Lunch	Snack	Dinner	Snack	Bedtime	Night	Notes
Blood Sugar									
Insulin Dose									
Grams Carb									
Activity									

Date:	Breakfast	Snack	Lunch	Snack	Dinner	Snack	Bedtime	Night	Notes
Blood Sugar									
Insulin Dose									
Grams Carb									
Activity									

Weekly Diabetes Record

Name: ______________________________

Date:	Breakfast	Snack	Lunch	Snack	Dinner	Snack	Bedtime	Night	Notes
Blood Sugar									
Insulin Dose									
Grams Carb									
Activity									

Date:	Breakfast	Snack	Lunch	Snack	Dinner	Snack	Bedtime	Night	Notes
Blood Sugar									
Insulin Dose									
Grams Carb									
Activity									

Date:	Breakfast	Snack	Lunch	Snack	Dinner	Snack	Bedtime	Night	Notes
Blood Sugar									
Insulin Dose									
Grams Carb									
Activity									

Date:	Breakfast	Snack	Lunch	Snack	Dinner	Snack	Bedtime	Night	Notes
Blood Sugar									
Insulin Dose									
Grams Carb									
Activity									

Date:	Breakfast	Snack	Lunch	Snack	Dinner	Snack	Bedtime	Night	Notes
Blood Sugar									
Insulin Dose									
Grams Carb									
Activity									

Date:	Breakfast	Snack	Lunch	Snack	Dinner	Snack	Bedtime	Night	Notes
Blood Sugar									
Insulin Dose									
Grams Carb									
Activity									

Date:	Breakfast	Snack	Lunch	Snack	Dinner	Snack	Bedtime	Night	Notes
Blood Sugar									
Insulin Dose									
Grams Carb									
Activity									

Weekly Diabetes Record

Name: ______________________________

Date:	Breakfast	Snack	Lunch	Snack	Dinner	Snack	Bedtime	Night	Notes
Blood Sugar									
Insulin Dose									
Grams Carb									
Activity									

Date:	Breakfast	Snack	Lunch	Snack	Dinner	Snack	Bedtime	Night	Notes
Blood Sugar									
Insulin Dose									
Grams Carb									
Activity									

Date:	Breakfast	Snack	Lunch	Snack	Dinner	Snack	Bedtime	Night	Notes
Blood Sugar									
Insulin Dose									
Grams Carb									
Activity									

Date:	Breakfast	Snack	Lunch	Snack	Dinner	Snack	Bedtime	Night	Notes
Blood Sugar									
Insulin Dose									
Grams Carb									
Activity									

Date:	Breakfast	Snack	Lunch	Snack	Dinner	Snack	Bedtime	Night	Notes
Blood Sugar									
Insulin Dose									
Grams Carb									
Activity									

Date:	Breakfast	Snack	Lunch	Snack	Dinner	Snack	Bedtime	Night	Notes
Blood Sugar									
Insulin Dose									
Grams Carb									
Activity									

Date:	Breakfast	Snack	Lunch	Snack	Dinner	Snack	Bedtime	Night	Notes
Blood Sugar									
Insulin Dose									
Grams Carb									
Activity									

Weekly Diabetes Record

Name: ______________________________

Date:	Breakfast	Snack	Lunch	Snack	Dinner	Snack	Bedtime	Night	Notes
Blood Sugar									
Insulin Dose									
Grams Carb									
Activity									

Date:	Breakfast	Snack	Lunch	Snack	Dinner	Snack	Bedtime	Night	Notes
Blood Sugar									
Insulin Dose									
Grams Carb									
Activity									

Date:	Breakfast	Snack	Lunch	Snack	Dinner	Snack	Bedtime	Night	Notes
Blood Sugar									
Insulin Dose									
Grams Carb									
Activity									

Date:	Breakfast	Snack	Lunch	Snack	Dinner	Snack	Bedtime	Night	Notes
Blood Sugar									
Insulin Dose									
Grams Carb									
Activity									

Date:	Breakfast	Snack	Lunch	Snack	Dinner	Snack	Bedtime	Night	Notes
Blood Sugar									
Insulin Dose									
Grams Carb									
Activity									

Date:	Breakfast	Snack	Lunch	Snack	Dinner	Snack	Bedtime	Night	Notes
Blood Sugar									
Insulin Dose									
Grams Carb									
Activity									

Date:	Breakfast	Snack	Lunch	Snack	Dinner	Snack	Bedtime	Night	Notes
Blood Sugar									
Insulin Dose									
Grams Carb									
Activity									

Weekly Diabetes Record

Name: ______________________________

Date:	Breakfast	Snack	Lunch	Snack	Dinner	Snack	Bedtime	Night	Notes
Blood Sugar									
Insulin Dose									
Grams Carb									
Activity									

Date:	Breakfast	Snack	Lunch	Snack	Dinner	Snack	Bedtime	Night	Notes
Blood Sugar									
Insulin Dose									
Grams Carb									
Activity									

Date:	Breakfast	Snack	Lunch	Snack	Dinner	Snack	Bedtime	Night	Notes
Blood Sugar									
Insulin Dose									
Grams Carb									
Activity									

Date:	Breakfast	Snack	Lunch	Snack	Dinner	Snack	Bedtime	Night	Notes
Blood Sugar									
Insulin Dose									
Grams Carb									
Activity									

Date:	Breakfast	Snack	Lunch	Snack	Dinner	Snack	Bedtime	Night	Notes
Blood Sugar									
Insulin Dose									
Grams Carb									
Activity									

Date:	Breakfast	Snack	Lunch	Snack	Dinner	Snack	Bedtime	Night	Notes
Blood Sugar									
Insulin Dose									
Grams Carb									
Activity									

Date:	Breakfast	Snack	Lunch	Snack	Dinner	Snack	Bedtime	Night	Notes
Blood Sugar									
Insulin Dose									
Grams Carb									
Activity									

Weekly Diabetes Record

Name: ______________________________

Date:	Breakfast	Snack	Lunch	Snack	Dinner	Snack	Bedtime	Night	Notes
Blood Sugar									
Insulin Dose									
Grams Carb									
Activity									

Date:	Breakfast	Snack	Lunch	Snack	Dinner	Snack	Bedtime	Night	Notes
Blood Sugar									
Insulin Dose									
Grams Carb									
Activity									

Date:	Breakfast	Snack	Lunch	Snack	Dinner	Snack	Bedtime	Night	Notes
Blood Sugar									
Insulin Dose									
Grams Carb									
Activity									

Date:	Breakfast	Snack	Lunch	Snack	Dinner	Snack	Bedtime	Night	Notes
Blood Sugar									
Insulin Dose									
Grams Carb									
Activity									

Date:	Breakfast	Snack	Lunch	Snack	Dinner	Snack	Bedtime	Night	Notes
Blood Sugar									
Insulin Dose									
Grams Carb									
Activity									

Date:	Breakfast	Snack	Lunch	Snack	Dinner	Snack	Bedtime	Night	Notes
Blood Sugar									
Insulin Dose									
Grams Carb									
Activity									

Date:	Breakfast	Snack	Lunch	Snack	Dinner	Snack	Bedtime	Night	Notes
Blood Sugar									
Insulin Dose									
Grams Carb									
Activity									

Weekly Diabetes Record

Name: ______________________________

Date:	Breakfast	Snack	Lunch	Snack	Dinner	Snack	Bedtime	Night	Notes
Blood Sugar									
Insulin Dose									
Grams Carb									
Activity									

Date:	Breakfast	Snack	Lunch	Snack	Dinner	Snack	Bedtime	Night	Notes
Blood Sugar									
Insulin Dose									
Grams Carb									
Activity									

Date:	Breakfast	Snack	Lunch	Snack	Dinner	Snack	Bedtime	Night	Notes
Blood Sugar									
Insulin Dose									
Grams Carb									
Activity									

Date:	Breakfast	Snack	Lunch	Snack	Dinner	Snack	Bedtime	Night	Notes
Blood Sugar									
Insulin Dose									
Grams Carb									
Activity									

Date:	Breakfast	Snack	Lunch	Snack	Dinner	Snack	Bedtime	Night	Notes
Blood Sugar									
Insulin Dose									
Grams Carb									
Activity									

Date:	Breakfast	Snack	Lunch	Snack	Dinner	Snack	Bedtime	Night	Notes
Blood Sugar									
Insulin Dose									
Grams Carb									
Activity									

Date:	Breakfast	Snack	Lunch	Snack	Dinner	Snack	Bedtime	Night	Notes
Blood Sugar									
Insulin Dose									
Grams Carb									
Activity									

Weekly Diabetes Record

Name: ______________________________

Date:	Breakfast	Snack	Lunch	Snack	Dinner	Snack	Bedtime	Night	Notes
Blood Sugar									
Insulin Dose									
Grams Carb									
Activity									

Date:	Breakfast	Snack	Lunch	Snack	Dinner	Snack	Bedtime	Night	Notes
Blood Sugar									
Insulin Dose									
Grams Carb									
Activity									

Date:	Breakfast	Snack	Lunch	Snack	Dinner	Snack	Bedtime	Night	Notes
Blood Sugar									
Insulin Dose									
Grams Carb									
Activity									

Date:	Breakfast	Snack	Lunch	Snack	Dinner	Snack	Bedtime	Night	Notes
Blood Sugar									
Insulin Dose									
Grams Carb									
Activity									

Date:	Breakfast	Snack	Lunch	Snack	Dinner	Snack	Bedtime	Night	Notes
Blood Sugar									
Insulin Dose									
Grams Carb									
Activity									

Date:	Breakfast	Snack	Lunch	Snack	Dinner	Snack	Bedtime	Night	Notes
Blood Sugar									
Insulin Dose									
Grams Carb									
Activity									

Date:	Breakfast	Snack	Lunch	Snack	Dinner	Snack	Bedtime	Night	Notes
Blood Sugar									
Insulin Dose									
Grams Carb									
Activity									

Weekly Diabetes Record

Name: ______________________________

Date:	Breakfast	Snack	Lunch	Snack	Dinner	Snack	Bedtime	Night	Notes
Blood Sugar									
Insulin Dose									
Grams Carb									
Activity									

Date:	Breakfast	Snack	Lunch	Snack	Dinner	Snack	Bedtime	Night	Notes
Blood Sugar									
Insulin Dose									
Grams Carb									
Activity									

Date:	Breakfast	Snack	Lunch	Snack	Dinner	Snack	Bedtime	Night	Notes
Blood Sugar									
Insulin Dose									
Grams Carb									
Activity									

Date:	Breakfast	Snack	Lunch	Snack	Dinner	Snack	Bedtime	Night	Notes
Blood Sugar									
Insulin Dose									
Grams Carb									
Activity									

Date:	Breakfast	Snack	Lunch	Snack	Dinner	Snack	Bedtime	Night	Notes
Blood Sugar									
Insulin Dose									
Grams Carb									
Activity									

Date:	Breakfast	Snack	Lunch	Snack	Dinner	Snack	Bedtime	Night	Notes
Blood Sugar									
Insulin Dose									
Grams Carb									
Activity									

Date:	Breakfast	Snack	Lunch	Snack	Dinner	Snack	Bedtime	Night	Notes
Blood Sugar									
Insulin Dose									
Grams Carb									
Activity									

Weekly Diabetes Record

Name: ______________________________

Date:	Breakfast	Snack	Lunch	Snack	Dinner	Snack	Bedtime	Night	Notes
Blood Sugar									
Insulin Dose									
Grams Carb									
Activity									

Date:	Breakfast	Snack	Lunch	Snack	Dinner	Snack	Bedtime	Night	Notes
Blood Sugar									
Insulin Dose									
Grams Carb									
Activity									

Date:	Breakfast	Snack	Lunch	Snack	Dinner	Snack	Bedtime	Night	Notes
Blood Sugar									
Insulin Dose									
Grams Carb									
Activity									

Date:	Breakfast	Snack	Lunch	Snack	Dinner	Snack	Bedtime	Night	Notes
Blood Sugar									
Insulin Dose									
Grams Carb									
Activity									

Date:	Breakfast	Snack	Lunch	Snack	Dinner	Snack	Bedtime	Night	Notes
Blood Sugar									
Insulin Dose									
Grams Carb									
Activity									

Date:	Breakfast	Snack	Lunch	Snack	Dinner	Snack	Bedtime	Night	Notes
Blood Sugar									
Insulin Dose									
Grams Carb									
Activity									

Date:	Breakfast	Snack	Lunch	Snack	Dinner	Snack	Bedtime	Night	Notes
Blood Sugar									
Insulin Dose									
Grams Carb									
Activity									

Weekly Diabetes Record

Name: ____

Date:	Breakfast	Snack	Lunch	Snack	Dinner	Snack	Bedtime	Night	Notes
Blood Sugar									
Insulin Dose									
Grams Carb									
Activity									

Date:	Breakfast	Snack	Lunch	Snack	Dinner	Snack	Bedtime	Night	Notes
Blood Sugar									
Insulin Dose									
Grams Carb									
Activity									

Date:	Breakfast	Snack	Lunch	Snack	Dinner	Snack	Bedtime	Night	Notes
Blood Sugar									
Insulin Dose									
Grams Carb									
Activity									

Date:	Breakfast	Snack	Lunch	Snack	Dinner	Snack	Bedtime	Night	Notes
Blood Sugar									
Insulin Dose									
Grams Carb									
Activity									

Date:	Breakfast	Snack	Lunch	Snack	Dinner	Snack	Bedtime	Night	Notes
Blood Sugar									
Insulin Dose									
Grams Carb									
Activity									

Date:	Breakfast	Snack	Lunch	Snack	Dinner	Snack	Bedtime	Night	Notes
Blood Sugar									
Insulin Dose									
Grams Carb									
Activity									

Date:	Breakfast	Snack	Lunch	Snack	Dinner	Snack	Bedtime	Night	Notes
Blood Sugar									
Insulin Dose									
Grams Carb									
Activity									

Weekly Diabetes Record

Name: ____________________

Date:	Breakfast	Snack	Lunch	Snack	Dinner	Snack	Bedtime	Night	Notes
Blood Sugar									
Insulin Dose									
Grams Carb									
Activity									

Date:	Breakfast	Snack	Lunch	Snack	Dinner	Snack	Bedtime	Night	Notes
Blood Sugar									
Insulin Dose									
Grams Carb									
Activity									

Date:	Breakfast	Snack	Lunch	Snack	Dinner	Snack	Bedtime	Night	Notes
Blood Sugar									
Insulin Dose									
Grams Carb									
Activity									

Date:	Breakfast	Snack	Lunch	Snack	Dinner	Snack	Bedtime	Night	Notes
Blood Sugar									
Insulin Dose									
Grams Carb									
Activity									

Date:	Breakfast	Snack	Lunch	Snack	Dinner	Snack	Bedtime	Night	Notes
Blood Sugar									
Insulin Dose									
Grams Carb									
Activity									

Date:	Breakfast	Snack	Lunch	Snack	Dinner	Snack	Bedtime	Night	Notes
Blood Sugar									
Insulin Dose									
Grams Carb									
Activity									

Date:	Breakfast	Snack	Lunch	Snack	Dinner	Snack	Bedtime	Night	Notes
Blood Sugar									
Insulin Dose									
Grams Carb									
Activity									

Weekly Diabetes Record

Name: ______________________________

Date:	Breakfast	Snack	Lunch	Snack	Dinner	Snack	Bedtime	Night	Notes
Blood Sugar									
Insulin Dose									
Grams Carb									
Activity									

Date:	Breakfast	Snack	Lunch	Snack	Dinner	Snack	Bedtime	Night	Notes
Blood Sugar									
Insulin Dose									
Grams Carb									
Activity									

Date:	Breakfast	Snack	Lunch	Snack	Dinner	Snack	Bedtime	Night	Notes
Blood Sugar									
Insulin Dose									
Grams Carb									
Activity									

Date:	Breakfast	Snack	Lunch	Snack	Dinner	Snack	Bedtime	Night	Notes
Blood Sugar									
Insulin Dose									
Grams Carb									
Activity									

Date:	Breakfast	Snack	Lunch	Snack	Dinner	Snack	Bedtime	Night	Notes
Blood Sugar									
Insulin Dose									
Grams Carb									
Activity									

Date:	Breakfast	Snack	Lunch	Snack	Dinner	Snack	Bedtime	Night	Notes
Blood Sugar									
Insulin Dose									
Grams Carb									
Activity									

Date:	Breakfast	Snack	Lunch	Snack	Dinner	Snack	Bedtime	Night	Notes
Blood Sugar									
Insulin Dose									
Grams Carb									
Activity									

Weekly Diabetes Record

Name: ________________________________

Date:	Breakfast	Snack	Lunch	Snack	Dinner	Snack	Bedtime	Night	Notes
Blood Sugar									
Insulin Dose									
Grams Carb									
Activity									

Date:	Breakfast	Snack	Lunch	Snack	Dinner	Snack	Bedtime	Night	Notes
Blood Sugar									
Insulin Dose									
Grams Carb									
Activity									

Date:	Breakfast	Snack	Lunch	Snack	Dinner	Snack	Bedtime	Night	Notes
Blood Sugar									
Insulin Dose									
Grams Carb									
Activity									

Date:	Breakfast	Snack	Lunch	Snack	Dinner	Snack	Bedtime	Night	Notes
Blood Sugar									
Insulin Dose									
Grams Carb									
Activity									

Date:	Breakfast	Snack	Lunch	Snack	Dinner	Snack	Bedtime	Night	Notes
Blood Sugar									
Insulin Dose									
Grams Carb									
Activity									

Date:	Breakfast	Snack	Lunch	Snack	Dinner	Snack	Bedtime	Night	Notes
Blood Sugar									
Insulin Dose									
Grams Carb									
Activity									

Date:	Breakfast	Snack	Lunch	Snack	Dinner	Snack	Bedtime	Night	Notes
Blood Sugar									
Insulin Dose									
Grams Carb									
Activity									

Weekly Diabetes Record

Name: ____

Date:	Breakfast	Snack	Lunch	Snack	Dinner	Snack	Bedtime	Night	Notes
Blood Sugar									
Insulin Dose									
Grams Carb									
Activity									

Date:	Breakfast	Snack	Lunch	Snack	Dinner	Snack	Bedtime	Night	Notes
Blood Sugar									
Insulin Dose									
Grams Carb									
Activity									

Date:	Breakfast	Snack	Lunch	Snack	Dinner	Snack	Bedtime	Night	Notes
Blood Sugar									
Insulin Dose									
Grams Carb									
Activity									

Date:	Breakfast	Snack	Lunch	Snack	Dinner	Snack	Bedtime	Night	Notes
Blood Sugar									
Insulin Dose									
Grams Carb									
Activity									

Date:	Breakfast	Snack	Lunch	Snack	Dinner	Snack	Bedtime	Night	Notes
Blood Sugar									
Insulin Dose									
Grams Carb									
Activity									

Date:	Breakfast	Snack	Lunch	Snack	Dinner	Snack	Bedtime	Night	Notes
Blood Sugar									
Insulin Dose									
Grams Carb									
Activity									

Date:	Breakfast	Snack	Lunch	Snack	Dinner	Snack	Bedtime	Night	Notes
Blood Sugar									
Insulin Dose									
Grams Carb									
Activity									

Weekly Diabetes Record

Name: ______________________________

Date:	Breakfast	Snack	Lunch	Snack	Dinner	Snack	Bedtime	Night	Notes
Blood Sugar									
Insulin Dose									
Grams Carb									
Activity									

Date:	Breakfast	Snack	Lunch	Snack	Dinner	Snack	Bedtime	Night	Notes
Blood Sugar									
Insulin Dose									
Grams Carb									
Activity									

Date:	Breakfast	Snack	Lunch	Snack	Dinner	Snack	Bedtime	Night	Notes
Blood Sugar									
Insulin Dose									
Grams Carb									
Activity									

Date:	Breakfast	Snack	Lunch	Snack	Dinner	Snack	Bedtime	Night	Notes
Blood Sugar									
Insulin Dose									
Grams Carb									
Activity									

Date:	Breakfast	Snack	Lunch	Snack	Dinner	Snack	Bedtime	Night	Notes
Blood Sugar									
Insulin Dose									
Grams Carb									
Activity									

Date:	Breakfast	Snack	Lunch	Snack	Dinner	Snack	Bedtime	Night	Notes
Blood Sugar									
Insulin Dose									
Grams Carb									
Activity									

Date:	Breakfast	Snack	Lunch	Snack	Dinner	Snack	Bedtime	Night	Notes
Blood Sugar									
Insulin Dose									
Grams Carb									
Activity									

Weekly Diabetes Record

Name: ____________________

Date:	Breakfast	Snack	Lunch	Snack	Dinner	Snack	Bedtime	Night	Notes
Blood Sugar									
Insulin Dose									
Grams Carb									
Activity									

Date:	Breakfast	Snack	Lunch	Snack	Dinner	Snack	Bedtime	Night	Notes
Blood Sugar									
Insulin Dose									
Grams Carb									
Activity									

Date:	Breakfast	Snack	Lunch	Snack	Dinner	Snack	Bedtime	Night	Notes
Blood Sugar									
Insulin Dose									
Grams Carb									
Activity									

Date:	Breakfast	Snack	Lunch	Snack	Dinner	Snack	Bedtime	Night	Notes
Blood Sugar									
Insulin Dose									
Grams Carb									
Activity									

Date:	Breakfast	Snack	Lunch	Snack	Dinner	Snack	Bedtime	Night	Notes
Blood Sugar									
Insulin Dose									
Grams Carb									
Activity									

Date:	Breakfast	Snack	Lunch	Snack	Dinner	Snack	Bedtime	Night	Notes
Blood Sugar									
Insulin Dose									
Grams Carb									
Activity									

Date:	Breakfast	Snack	Lunch	Snack	Dinner	Snack	Bedtime	Night	Notes
Blood Sugar									
Insulin Dose									
Grams Carb									
Activity									

Weekly Diabetes Record

Name: ____________________________________

Date:	Breakfast	Snack	Lunch	Snack	Dinner	Snack	Bedtime	Night	Notes
Blood Sugar									
Insulin Dose									
Grams Carb									
Activity									

Date:	Breakfast	Snack	Lunch	Snack	Dinner	Snack	Bedtime	Night	Notes
Blood Sugar									
Insulin Dose									
Grams Carb									
Activity									

Date:	Breakfast	Snack	Lunch	Snack	Dinner	Snack	Bedtime	Night	Notes
Blood Sugar									
Insulin Dose									
Grams Carb									
Activity									

Date:	Breakfast	Snack	Lunch	Snack	Dinner	Snack	Bedtime	Night	Notes
Blood Sugar									
Insulin Dose									
Grams Carb									
Activity									

Date:	Breakfast	Snack	Lunch	Snack	Dinner	Snack	Bedtime	Night	Notes
Blood Sugar									
Insulin Dose									
Grams Carb									
Activity									

Date:	Breakfast	Snack	Lunch	Snack	Dinner	Snack	Bedtime	Night	Notes
Blood Sugar									
Insulin Dose									
Grams Carb									
Activity									

Date:	Breakfast	Snack	Lunch	Snack	Dinner	Snack	Bedtime	Night	Notes
Blood Sugar									
Insulin Dose									
Grams Carb									
Activity									

Weekly Diabetes Record

Name: ______________________________

Date:	Breakfast	Snack	Lunch	Snack	Dinner	Snack	Bedtime	Night	Notes
Blood Sugar									
Insulin Dose									
Grams Carb									
Activity									

Date:	Breakfast	Snack	Lunch	Snack	Dinner	Snack	Bedtime	Night	Notes
Blood Sugar									
Insulin Dose									
Grams Carb									
Activity									

Date:	Breakfast	Snack	Lunch	Snack	Dinner	Snack	Bedtime	Night	Notes
Blood Sugar									
Insulin Dose									
Grams Carb									
Activity									

Date:	Breakfast	Snack	Lunch	Snack	Dinner	Snack	Bedtime	Night	Notes
Blood Sugar									
Insulin Dose									
Grams Carb									
Activity									

Date:	Breakfast	Snack	Lunch	Snack	Dinner	Snack	Bedtime	Night	Notes
Blood Sugar									
Insulin Dose									
Grams Carb									
Activity									

Date:	Breakfast	Snack	Lunch	Snack	Dinner	Snack	Bedtime	Night	Notes
Blood Sugar									
Insulin Dose									
Grams Carb									
Activity									

Date:	Breakfast	Snack	Lunch	Snack	Dinner	Snack	Bedtime	Night	Notes
Blood Sugar									
Insulin Dose									
Grams Carb									
Activity									

Weekly Diabetes Record

Name: ______________________________

Date:	Breakfast	Snack	Lunch	Snack	Dinner	Snack	Bedtime	Night	Notes
Blood Sugar									
Insulin Dose									
Grams Carb									
Activity									

Date:	Breakfast	Snack	Lunch	Snack	Dinner	Snack	Bedtime	Night	Notes
Blood Sugar									
Insulin Dose									
Grams Carb									
Activity									

Date:	Breakfast	Snack	Lunch	Snack	Dinner	Snack	Bedtime	Night	Notes
Blood Sugar									
Insulin Dose									
Grams Carb									
Activity									

Date:	Breakfast	Snack	Lunch	Snack	Dinner	Snack	Bedtime	Night	Notes
Blood Sugar									
Insulin Dose									
Grams Carb									
Activity									

Date:	Breakfast	Snack	Lunch	Snack	Dinner	Snack	Bedtime	Night	Notes
Blood Sugar									
Insulin Dose									
Grams Carb									
Activity									

Date:	Breakfast	Snack	Lunch	Snack	Dinner	Snack	Bedtime	Night	Notes
Blood Sugar									
Insulin Dose									
Grams Carb									
Activity									

Date:	Breakfast	Snack	Lunch	Snack	Dinner	Snack	Bedtime	Night	Notes
Blood Sugar									
Insulin Dose									
Grams Carb									
Activity									

Weekly Diabetes Record

Name: ______________________________

Date:	Breakfast	Snack	Lunch	Snack	Dinner	Snack	Bedtime	Night	Notes
Blood Sugar									
Insulin Dose									
Grams Carb									
Activity									

Date:	Breakfast	Snack	Lunch	Snack	Dinner	Snack	Bedtime	Night	Notes
Blood Sugar									
Insulin Dose									
Grams Carb									
Activity									

Date:	Breakfast	Snack	Lunch	Snack	Dinner	Snack	Bedtime	Night	Notes
Blood Sugar									
Insulin Dose									
Grams Carb									
Activity									

Date:	Breakfast	Snack	Lunch	Snack	Dinner	Snack	Bedtime	Night	Notes
Blood Sugar									
Insulin Dose									
Grams Carb									
Activity									

Date:	Breakfast	Snack	Lunch	Snack	Dinner	Snack	Bedtime	Night	Notes
Blood Sugar									
Insulin Dose									
Grams Carb									
Activity									

Date:	Breakfast	Snack	Lunch	Snack	Dinner	Snack	Bedtime	Night	Notes
Blood Sugar									
Insulin Dose									
Grams Carb									
Activity									

Date:	Breakfast	Snack	Lunch	Snack	Dinner	Snack	Bedtime	Night	Notes
Blood Sugar									
Insulin Dose									
Grams Carb									
Activity									

Weekly Diabetes Record

Name: ______________________________

Date:	Breakfast	Snack	Lunch	Snack	Dinner	Snack	Bedtime	Night	Notes
Blood Sugar									
Insulin Dose									
Grams Carb									
Activity									

Date:	Breakfast	Snack	Lunch	Snack	Dinner	Snack	Bedtime	Night	Notes
Blood Sugar									
Insulin Dose									
Grams Carb									
Activity									

Date:	Breakfast	Snack	Lunch	Snack	Dinner	Snack	Bedtime	Night	Notes
Blood Sugar									
Insulin Dose									
Grams Carb									
Activity									

Date:	Breakfast	Snack	Lunch	Snack	Dinner	Snack	Bedtime	Night	Notes
Blood Sugar									
Insulin Dose									
Grams Carb									
Activity									

Date:	Breakfast	Snack	Lunch	Snack	Dinner	Snack	Bedtime	Night	Notes
Blood Sugar									
Insulin Dose									
Grams Carb									
Activity									

Date:	Breakfast	Snack	Lunch	Snack	Dinner	Snack	Bedtime	Night	Notes
Blood Sugar									
Insulin Dose									
Grams Carb									
Activity									

Date:	Breakfast	Snack	Lunch	Snack	Dinner	Snack	Bedtime	Night	Notes
Blood Sugar									
Insulin Dose									
Grams Carb									
Activity									

Weekly Diabetes Record

Name: ______________________________

Date:	Breakfast	Snack	Lunch	Snack	Dinner	Snack	Bedtime	Night	Notes
Blood Sugar									
Insulin Dose									
Grams Carb									
Activity									

Date:	Breakfast	Snack	Lunch	Snack	Dinner	Snack	Bedtime	Night	Notes
Blood Sugar									
Insulin Dose									
Grams Carb									
Activity									

Date:	Breakfast	Snack	Lunch	Snack	Dinner	Snack	Bedtime	Night	Notes
Blood Sugar									
Insulin Dose									
Grams Carb									
Activity									

Date:	Breakfast	Snack	Lunch	Snack	Dinner	Snack	Bedtime	Night	Notes
Blood Sugar									
Insulin Dose									
Grams Carb									
Activity									

Date:	Breakfast	Snack	Lunch	Snack	Dinner	Snack	Bedtime	Night	Notes
Blood Sugar									
Insulin Dose									
Grams Carb									
Activity									

Date:	Breakfast	Snack	Lunch	Snack	Dinner	Snack	Bedtime	Night	Notes
Blood Sugar									
Insulin Dose									
Grams Carb									
Activity									

Date:	Breakfast	Snack	Lunch	Snack	Dinner	Snack	Bedtime	Night	Notes
Blood Sugar									
Insulin Dose									
Grams Carb									
Activity									

Weekly Diabetes Record

Name: ______________________________

Date:	Breakfast	Snack	Lunch	Snack	Dinner	Snack	Bedtime	Night	Notes
Blood Sugar									
Insulin Dose									
Grams Carb									
Activity									

Date:	Breakfast	Snack	Lunch	Snack	Dinner	Snack	Bedtime	Night	Notes
Blood Sugar									
Insulin Dose									
Grams Carb									
Activity									

Date:	Breakfast	Snack	Lunch	Snack	Dinner	Snack	Bedtime	Night	Notes
Blood Sugar									
Insulin Dose									
Grams Carb									
Activity									

Date:	Breakfast	Snack	Lunch	Snack	Dinner	Snack	Bedtime	Night	Notes
Blood Sugar									
Insulin Dose									
Grams Carb									
Activity									

Date:	Breakfast	Snack	Lunch	Snack	Dinner	Snack	Bedtime	Night	Notes
Blood Sugar									
Insulin Dose									
Grams Carb									
Activity									

Date:	Breakfast	Snack	Lunch	Snack	Dinner	Snack	Bedtime	Night	Notes
Blood Sugar									
Insulin Dose									
Grams Carb									
Activity									

Date:	Breakfast	Snack	Lunch	Snack	Dinner	Snack	Bedtime	Night	Notes
Blood Sugar									
Insulin Dose									
Grams Carb									
Activity									

Weekly Diabetes Record

Name: ______________________________

Date:	Breakfast	Snack	Lunch	Snack	Dinner	Snack	Bedtime	Night	Notes
Blood Sugar									
Insulin Dose									
Grams Carb									
Activity									

Date:	Breakfast	Snack	Lunch	Snack	Dinner	Snack	Bedtime	Night	Notes
Blood Sugar									
Insulin Dose									
Grams Carb									
Activity									

Date:	Breakfast	Snack	Lunch	Snack	Dinner	Snack	Bedtime	Night	Notes
Blood Sugar									
Insulin Dose									
Grams Carb									
Activity									

Date:	Breakfast	Snack	Lunch	Snack	Dinner	Snack	Bedtime	Night	Notes
Blood Sugar									
Insulin Dose									
Grams Carb									
Activity									

Date:	Breakfast	Snack	Lunch	Snack	Dinner	Snack	Bedtime	Night	Notes
Blood Sugar									
Insulin Dose									
Grams Carb									
Activity									

Date:	Breakfast	Snack	Lunch	Snack	Dinner	Snack	Bedtime	Night	Notes
Blood Sugar									
Insulin Dose									
Grams Carb									
Activity									

Date:	Breakfast	Snack	Lunch	Snack	Dinner	Snack	Bedtime	Night	Notes
Blood Sugar									
Insulin Dose									
Grams Carb									
Activity									

Weekly Diabetes Record

Name: ________________________________

Date:	Breakfast	Snack	Lunch	Snack	Dinner	Snack	Bedtime	Night	Notes
Blood Sugar									
Insulin Dose									
Grams Carb									
Activity									

Date:	Breakfast	Snack	Lunch	Snack	Dinner	Snack	Bedtime	Night	Notes
Blood Sugar									
Insulin Dose									
Grams Carb									
Activity									

Date:	Breakfast	Snack	Lunch	Snack	Dinner	Snack	Bedtime	Night	Notes
Blood Sugar									
Insulin Dose									
Grams Carb									
Activity									

Date:	Breakfast	Snack	Lunch	Snack	Dinner	Snack	Bedtime	Night	Notes
Blood Sugar									
Insulin Dose									
Grams Carb									
Activity									

Date:	Breakfast	Snack	Lunch	Snack	Dinner	Snack	Bedtime	Night	Notes
Blood Sugar									
Insulin Dose									
Grams Carb									
Activity									

Date:	Breakfast	Snack	Lunch	Snack	Dinner	Snack	Bedtime	Night	Notes
Blood Sugar									
Insulin Dose									
Grams Carb									
Activity									

Date:	Breakfast	Snack	Lunch	Snack	Dinner	Snack	Bedtime	Night	Notes
Blood Sugar									
Insulin Dose									
Grams Carb									
Activity									

Weekly Diabetes Record

Name: ______________________________

Date:	Breakfast	Snack	Lunch	Snack	Dinner	Snack	Bedtime	Night	Notes
Blood Sugar									
Insulin Dose									
Grams Carb									
Activity									

Date:	Breakfast	Snack	Lunch	Snack	Dinner	Snack	Bedtime	Night	Notes
Blood Sugar									
Insulin Dose									
Grams Carb									
Activity									

Date:	Breakfast	Snack	Lunch	Snack	Dinner	Snack	Bedtime	Night	Notes
Blood Sugar									
Insulin Dose									
Grams Carb									
Activity									

Date:	Breakfast	Snack	Lunch	Snack	Dinner	Snack	Bedtime	Night	Notes
Blood Sugar									
Insulin Dose									
Grams Carb									
Activity									

Date:	Breakfast	Snack	Lunch	Snack	Dinner	Snack	Bedtime	Night	Notes
Blood Sugar									
Insulin Dose									
Grams Carb									
Activity									

Date:	Breakfast	Snack	Lunch	Snack	Dinner	Snack	Bedtime	Night	Notes
Blood Sugar									
Insulin Dose									
Grams Carb									
Activity									

Date:	Breakfast	Snack	Lunch	Snack	Dinner	Snack	Bedtime	Night	Notes
Blood Sugar									
Insulin Dose									
Grams Carb									
Activity									

Weekly Diabetes Record

Name: ____

Date:	Breakfast	Snack	Lunch	Snack	Dinner	Snack	Bedtime	Night	Notes
Blood Sugar									
Insulin Dose									
Grams Carb									
Activity									

Date:	Breakfast	Snack	Lunch	Snack	Dinner	Snack	Bedtime	Night	Notes
Blood Sugar									
Insulin Dose									
Grams Carb									
Activity									

Date:	Breakfast	Snack	Lunch	Snack	Dinner	Snack	Bedtime	Night	Notes
Blood Sugar									
Insulin Dose									
Grams Carb									
Activity									

Date:	Breakfast	Snack	Lunch	Snack	Dinner	Snack	Bedtime	Night	Notes
Blood Sugar									
Insulin Dose									
Grams Carb									
Activity									

Date:	Breakfast	Snack	Lunch	Snack	Dinner	Snack	Bedtime	Night	Notes
Blood Sugar									
Insulin Dose									
Grams Carb									
Activity									

Date:	Breakfast	Snack	Lunch	Snack	Dinner	Snack	Bedtime	Night	Notes
Blood Sugar									
Insulin Dose									
Grams Carb									
Activity									

Date:	Breakfast	Snack	Lunch	Snack	Dinner	Snack	Bedtime	Night	Notes
Blood Sugar									
Insulin Dose									
Grams Carb									
Activity									

Weekly Diabetes Record

Name: ______________________________

Date:	Breakfast	Snack	Lunch	Snack	Dinner	Snack	Bedtime	Night	Notes
Blood Sugar									
Insulin Dose									
Grams Carb									
Activity									

Date:	Breakfast	Snack	Lunch	Snack	Dinner	Snack	Bedtime	Night	Notes
Blood Sugar									
Insulin Dose									
Grams Carb									
Activity									

Date:	Breakfast	Snack	Lunch	Snack	Dinner	Snack	Bedtime	Night	Notes
Blood Sugar									
Insulin Dose									
Grams Carb									
Activity									

Date:	Breakfast	Snack	Lunch	Snack	Dinner	Snack	Bedtime	Night	Notes
Blood Sugar									
Insulin Dose									
Grams Carb									
Activity									

Date:	Breakfast	Snack	Lunch	Snack	Dinner	Snack	Bedtime	Night	Notes
Blood Sugar									
Insulin Dose									
Grams Carb									
Activity									

Date:	Breakfast	Snack	Lunch	Snack	Dinner	Snack	Bedtime	Night	Notes
Blood Sugar									
Insulin Dose									
Grams Carb									
Activity									

Date:	Breakfast	Snack	Lunch	Snack	Dinner	Snack	Bedtime	Night	Notes
Blood Sugar									
Insulin Dose									
Grams Carb									
Activity									

Weekly Diabetes Record

Name: ____

Date:	Breakfast	Snack	Lunch	Snack	Dinner	Snack	Bedtime	Night	Notes
Blood Sugar									
Insulin Dose									
Grams Carb									
Activity									

Date:	Breakfast	Snack	Lunch	Snack	Dinner	Snack	Bedtime	Night	Notes
Blood Sugar									
Insulin Dose									
Grams Carb									
Activity									

Date:	Breakfast	Snack	Lunch	Snack	Dinner	Snack	Bedtime	Night	Notes
Blood Sugar									
Insulin Dose									
Grams Carb									
Activity									

Date:	Breakfast	Snack	Lunch	Snack	Dinner	Snack	Bedtime	Night	Notes
Blood Sugar									
Insulin Dose									
Grams Carb									
Activity									

Date:	Breakfast	Snack	Lunch	Snack	Dinner	Snack	Bedtime	Night	Notes
Blood Sugar									
Insulin Dose									
Grams Carb									
Activity									

Date:	Breakfast	Snack	Lunch	Snack	Dinner	Snack	Bedtime	Night	Notes
Blood Sugar									
Insulin Dose									
Grams Carb									
Activity									

Date:	Breakfast	Snack	Lunch	Snack	Dinner	Snack	Bedtime	Night	Notes
Blood Sugar									
Insulin Dose									
Grams Carb									
Activity									

Weekly Diabetes Record

Name: ______________________________

Date:	Breakfast	Snack	Lunch	Snack	Dinner	Snack	Bedtime	Night	Notes
Blood Sugar									
Insulin Dose									
Grams Carb									
Activity									

Date:	Breakfast	Snack	Lunch	Snack	Dinner	Snack	Bedtime	Night	Notes
Blood Sugar									
Insulin Dose									
Grams Carb									
Activity									

Date:	Breakfast	Snack	Lunch	Snack	Dinner	Snack	Bedtime	Night	Notes
Blood Sugar									
Insulin Dose									
Grams Carb									
Activity									

Date:	Breakfast	Snack	Lunch	Snack	Dinner	Snack	Bedtime	Night	Notes
Blood Sugar									
Insulin Dose									
Grams Carb									
Activity									

Date:	Breakfast	Snack	Lunch	Snack	Dinner	Snack	Bedtime	Night	Notes
Blood Sugar									
Insulin Dose									
Grams Carb									
Activity									

Date:	Breakfast	Snack	Lunch	Snack	Dinner	Snack	Bedtime	Night	Notes
Blood Sugar									
Insulin Dose									
Grams Carb									
Activity									

Date:	Breakfast	Snack	Lunch	Snack	Dinner	Snack	Bedtime	Night	Notes
Blood Sugar									
Insulin Dose									
Grams Carb									
Activity									

Weekly Diabetes Record

Name: ______________________________

Date:	Breakfast	Snack	Lunch	Snack	Dinner	Snack	Bedtime	Night	Notes
Blood Sugar									
Insulin Dose									
Grams Carb									
Activity									

Date:	Breakfast	Snack	Lunch	Snack	Dinner	Snack	Bedtime	Night	Notes
Blood Sugar									
Insulin Dose									
Grams Carb									
Activity									

Date:	Breakfast	Snack	Lunch	Snack	Dinner	Snack	Bedtime	Night	Notes
Blood Sugar									
Insulin Dose									
Grams Carb									
Activity									

Date:	Breakfast	Snack	Lunch	Snack	Dinner	Snack	Bedtime	Night	Notes
Blood Sugar									
Insulin Dose									
Grams Carb									
Activity									

Date:	Breakfast	Snack	Lunch	Snack	Dinner	Snack	Bedtime	Night	Notes
Blood Sugar									
Insulin Dose									
Grams Carb									
Activity									

Date:	Breakfast	Snack	Lunch	Snack	Dinner	Snack	Bedtime	Night	Notes
Blood Sugar									
Insulin Dose									
Grams Carb									
Activity									

Date:	Breakfast	Snack	Lunch	Snack	Dinner	Snack	Bedtime	Night	Notes
Blood Sugar									
Insulin Dose									
Grams Carb									
Activity									

Weekly Diabetes Record

Name: ______________________________

Date:	Breakfast	Snack	Lunch	Snack	Dinner	Snack	Bedtime	Night	Notes
Blood Sugar									
Insulin Dose									
Grams Carb									
Activity									

Date:	Breakfast	Snack	Lunch	Snack	Dinner	Snack	Bedtime	Night	Notes
Blood Sugar									
Insulin Dose									
Grams Carb									
Activity									

Date:	Breakfast	Snack	Lunch	Snack	Dinner	Snack	Bedtime	Night	Notes
Blood Sugar									
Insulin Dose									
Grams Carb									
Activity									

Date:	Breakfast	Snack	Lunch	Snack	Dinner	Snack	Bedtime	Night	Notes
Blood Sugar									
Insulin Dose									
Grams Carb									
Activity									

Date:	Breakfast	Snack	Lunch	Snack	Dinner	Snack	Bedtime	Night	Notes
Blood Sugar									
Insulin Dose									
Grams Carb									
Activity									

Date:	Breakfast	Snack	Lunch	Snack	Dinner	Snack	Bedtime	Night	Notes
Blood Sugar									
Insulin Dose									
Grams Carb									
Activity									

Date:	Breakfast	Snack	Lunch	Snack	Dinner	Snack	Bedtime	Night	Notes
Blood Sugar									
Insulin Dose									
Grams Carb									
Activity									

Weekly Diabetes Record

Name: ______________________________

Date:	Breakfast	Snack	Lunch	Snack	Dinner	Snack	Bedtime	Night	Notes
Blood Sugar									
Insulin Dose									
Grams Carb									
Activity									

Date:	Breakfast	Snack	Lunch	Snack	Dinner	Snack	Bedtime	Night	Notes
Blood Sugar									
Insulin Dose									
Grams Carb									
Activity									

Date:	Breakfast	Snack	Lunch	Snack	Dinner	Snack	Bedtime	Night	Notes
Blood Sugar									
Insulin Dose									
Grams Carb									
Activity									

Date:	Breakfast	Snack	Lunch	Snack	Dinner	Snack	Bedtime	Night	Notes
Blood Sugar									
Insulin Dose									
Grams Carb									
Activity									

Date:	Breakfast	Snack	Lunch	Snack	Dinner	Snack	Bedtime	Night	Notes
Blood Sugar									
Insulin Dose									
Grams Carb									
Activity									

Date:	Breakfast	Snack	Lunch	Snack	Dinner	Snack	Bedtime	Night	Notes
Blood Sugar									
Insulin Dose									
Grams Carb									
Activity									

Date:	Breakfast	Snack	Lunch	Snack	Dinner	Snack	Bedtime	Night	Notes
Blood Sugar									
Insulin Dose									
Grams Carb									
Activity									

Weekly Diabetes Record

Name: ____________________

Date:	Breakfast	Snack	Lunch	Snack	Dinner	Snack	Bedtime	Night	Notes
Blood Sugar									
Insulin Dose									
Grams Carb									
Activity									

Date:	Breakfast	Snack	Lunch	Snack	Dinner	Snack	Bedtime	Night	Notes
Blood Sugar									
Insulin Dose									
Grams Carb									
Activity									

Date:	Breakfast	Snack	Lunch	Snack	Dinner	Snack	Bedtime	Night	Notes
Blood Sugar									
Insulin Dose									
Grams Carb									
Activity									

Date:	Breakfast	Snack	Lunch	Snack	Dinner	Snack	Bedtime	Night	Notes
Blood Sugar									
Insulin Dose									
Grams Carb									
Activity									

Date:	Breakfast	Snack	Lunch	Snack	Dinner	Snack	Bedtime	Night	Notes
Blood Sugar									
Insulin Dose									
Grams Carb									
Activity									

Date:	Breakfast	Snack	Lunch	Snack	Dinner	Snack	Bedtime	Night	Notes
Blood Sugar									
Insulin Dose									
Grams Carb									
Activity									

Date:	Breakfast	Snack	Lunch	Snack	Dinner	Snack	Bedtime	Night	Notes
Blood Sugar									
Insulin Dose									
Grams Carb									
Activity									

Weekly Diabetes Record

Name: ______________________________

Date:	Breakfast	Snack	Lunch	Snack	Dinner	Snack	Bedtime	Night	Notes
Blood Sugar									
Insulin Dose									
Grams Carb									
Activity									

Date:	Breakfast	Snack	Lunch	Snack	Dinner	Snack	Bedtime	Night	Notes
Blood Sugar									
Insulin Dose									
Grams Carb									
Activity									

Date:	Breakfast	Snack	Lunch	Snack	Dinner	Snack	Bedtime	Night	Notes
Blood Sugar									
Insulin Dose									
Grams Carb									
Activity									

Date:	Breakfast	Snack	Lunch	Snack	Dinner	Snack	Bedtime	Night	Notes
Blood Sugar									
Insulin Dose									
Grams Carb									
Activity									

Date:	Breakfast	Snack	Lunch	Snack	Dinner	Snack	Bedtime	Night	Notes
Blood Sugar									
Insulin Dose									
Grams Carb									
Activity									

Date:	Breakfast	Snack	Lunch	Snack	Dinner	Snack	Bedtime	Night	Notes
Blood Sugar									
Insulin Dose									
Grams Carb									
Activity									

Date:	Breakfast	Snack	Lunch	Snack	Dinner	Snack	Bedtime	Night	Notes
Blood Sugar									
Insulin Dose									
Grams Carb									
Activity									

Weekly Diabetes Record

Name: ______________________________

Date:	Breakfast	Snack	Lunch	Snack	Dinner	Snack	Bedtime	Night	Notes
Blood Sugar									
Insulin Dose									
Grams Carb									
Activity									

Date:	Breakfast	Snack	Lunch	Snack	Dinner	Snack	Bedtime	Night	Notes
Blood Sugar									
Insulin Dose									
Grams Carb									
Activity									

Date:	Breakfast	Snack	Lunch	Snack	Dinner	Snack	Bedtime	Night	Notes
Blood Sugar									
Insulin Dose									
Grams Carb									
Activity									

Date:	Breakfast	Snack	Lunch	Snack	Dinner	Snack	Bedtime	Night	Notes
Blood Sugar									
Insulin Dose									
Grams Carb									
Activity									

Date:	Breakfast	Snack	Lunch	Snack	Dinner	Snack	Bedtime	Night	Notes
Blood Sugar									
Insulin Dose									
Grams Carb									
Activity									

Date:	Breakfast	Snack	Lunch	Snack	Dinner	Snack	Bedtime	Night	Notes
Blood Sugar									
Insulin Dose									
Grams Carb									
Activity									

Date:	Breakfast	Snack	Lunch	Snack	Dinner	Snack	Bedtime	Night	Notes
Blood Sugar									
Insulin Dose									
Grams Carb									
Activity									

Weekly Diabetes Record

Name: ______________________________

Date:	Breakfast	Snack	Lunch	Snack	Dinner	Snack	Bedtime	Night	Notes
Blood Sugar									
Insulin Dose									
Grams Carb									
Activity									

Date:	Breakfast	Snack	Lunch	Snack	Dinner	Snack	Bedtime	Night	Notes
Blood Sugar									
Insulin Dose									
Grams Carb									
Activity									

Date:	Breakfast	Snack	Lunch	Snack	Dinner	Snack	Bedtime	Night	Notes
Blood Sugar									
Insulin Dose									
Grams Carb									
Activity									

Date:	Breakfast	Snack	Lunch	Snack	Dinner	Snack	Bedtime	Night	Notes
Blood Sugar									
Insulin Dose									
Grams Carb									
Activity									

Date:	Breakfast	Snack	Lunch	Snack	Dinner	Snack	Bedtime	Night	Notes
Blood Sugar									
Insulin Dose									
Grams Carb									
Activity									

Date:	Breakfast	Snack	Lunch	Snack	Dinner	Snack	Bedtime	Night	Notes
Blood Sugar									
Insulin Dose									
Grams Carb									
Activity									

Date:	Breakfast	Snack	Lunch	Snack	Dinner	Snack	Bedtime	Night	Notes
Blood Sugar									
Insulin Dose									
Grams Carb									
Activity									

Weekly Diabetes Record

Name: ______________________________

Date:	Breakfast	Snack	Lunch	Snack	Dinner	Snack	Bedtime	Night	Notes
Blood Sugar									
Insulin Dose									
Grams Carb									
Activity									

Date:	Breakfast	Snack	Lunch	Snack	Dinner	Snack	Bedtime	Night	Notes
Blood Sugar									
Insulin Dose									
Grams Carb									
Activity									

Date:	Breakfast	Snack	Lunch	Snack	Dinner	Snack	Bedtime	Night	Notes
Blood Sugar									
Insulin Dose									
Grams Carb									
Activity									

Date:	Breakfast	Snack	Lunch	Snack	Dinner	Snack	Bedtime	Night	Notes
Blood Sugar									
Insulin Dose									
Grams Carb									
Activity									

Date:	Breakfast	Snack	Lunch	Snack	Dinner	Snack	Bedtime	Night	Notes
Blood Sugar									
Insulin Dose									
Grams Carb									
Activity									

Date:	Breakfast	Snack	Lunch	Snack	Dinner	Snack	Bedtime	Night	Notes
Blood Sugar									
Insulin Dose									
Grams Carb									
Activity									

Date:	Breakfast	Snack	Lunch	Snack	Dinner	Snack	Bedtime	Night	Notes
Blood Sugar									
Insulin Dose									
Grams Carb									
Activity									

Weekly Diabetes Record

Name: ________________________________

Date:	Breakfast	Snack	Lunch	Snack	Dinner	Snack	Bedtime	Night	Notes
Blood Sugar									
Insulin Dose									
Grams Carb									
Activity									

Date:	Breakfast	Snack	Lunch	Snack	Dinner	Snack	Bedtime	Night	Notes
Blood Sugar									
Insulin Dose									
Grams Carb									
Activity									

Date:	Breakfast	Snack	Lunch	Snack	Dinner	Snack	Bedtime	Night	Notes
Blood Sugar									
Insulin Dose									
Grams Carb									
Activity									

Date:	Breakfast	Snack	Lunch	Snack	Dinner	Snack	Bedtime	Night	Notes
Blood Sugar									
Insulin Dose									
Grams Carb									
Activity									

Date:	Breakfast	Snack	Lunch	Snack	Dinner	Snack	Bedtime	Night	Notes
Blood Sugar									
Insulin Dose									
Grams Carb									
Activity									

Date:	Breakfast	Snack	Lunch	Snack	Dinner	Snack	Bedtime	Night	Notes
Blood Sugar									
Insulin Dose									
Grams Carb									
Activity									

Date:	Breakfast	Snack	Lunch	Snack	Dinner	Snack	Bedtime	Night	Notes
Blood Sugar									
Insulin Dose									
Grams Carb									
Activity									

Weekly Diabetes Record

Name: ______________________________

Date:	Breakfast	Snack	Lunch	Snack	Dinner	Snack	Bedtime	Night	Notes
Blood Sugar									
Insulin Dose									
Grams Carb									
Activity									

Date:	Breakfast	Snack	Lunch	Snack	Dinner	Snack	Bedtime	Night	Notes
Blood Sugar									
Insulin Dose									
Grams Carb									
Activity									

Date:	Breakfast	Snack	Lunch	Snack	Dinner	Snack	Bedtime	Night	Notes
Blood Sugar									
Insulin Dose									
Grams Carb									
Activity									

Date:	Breakfast	Snack	Lunch	Snack	Dinner	Snack	Bedtime	Night	Notes
Blood Sugar									
Insulin Dose									
Grams Carb									
Activity									

Date:	Breakfast	Snack	Lunch	Snack	Dinner	Snack	Bedtime	Night	Notes
Blood Sugar									
Insulin Dose									
Grams Carb									
Activity									

Date:	Breakfast	Snack	Lunch	Snack	Dinner	Snack	Bedtime	Night	Notes
Blood Sugar									
Insulin Dose									
Grams Carb									
Activity									

Date:	Breakfast	Snack	Lunch	Snack	Dinner	Snack	Bedtime	Night	Notes
Blood Sugar									
Insulin Dose									
Grams Carb									
Activity									

Weekly Diabetes Record

Name: ______________________________

Date:	Breakfast	Snack	Lunch	Snack	Dinner	Snack	Bedtime	Night	Notes
Blood Sugar									
Insulin Dose									
Grams Carb									
Activity									

Date:	Breakfast	Snack	Lunch	Snack	Dinner	Snack	Bedtime	Night	Notes
Blood Sugar									
Insulin Dose									
Grams Carb									
Activity									

Date:	Breakfast	Snack	Lunch	Snack	Dinner	Snack	Bedtime	Night	Notes
Blood Sugar									
Insulin Dose									
Grams Carb									
Activity									

Date:	Breakfast	Snack	Lunch	Snack	Dinner	Snack	Bedtime	Night	Notes
Blood Sugar									
Insulin Dose									
Grams Carb									
Activity									

Date:	Breakfast	Snack	Lunch	Snack	Dinner	Snack	Bedtime	Night	Notes
Blood Sugar									
Insulin Dose									
Grams Carb									
Activity									

Date:	Breakfast	Snack	Lunch	Snack	Dinner	Snack	Bedtime	Night	Notes
Blood Sugar									
Insulin Dose									
Grams Carb									
Activity									

Date:	Breakfast	Snack	Lunch	Snack	Dinner	Snack	Bedtime	Night	Notes
Blood Sugar									
Insulin Dose									
Grams Carb									
Activity									

Weekly Diabetes Record

Name: ____

Date:	Breakfast	Snack	Lunch	Snack	Dinner	Snack	Bedtime	Night	Notes
Blood Sugar									
Insulin Dose									
Grams Carb									
Activity									

Date:	Breakfast	Snack	Lunch	Snack	Dinner	Snack	Bedtime	Night	Notes
Blood Sugar									
Insulin Dose									
Grams Carb									
Activity									

Date:	Breakfast	Snack	Lunch	Snack	Dinner	Snack	Bedtime	Night	Notes
Blood Sugar									
Insulin Dose									
Grams Carb									
Activity									

Date:	Breakfast	Snack	Lunch	Snack	Dinner	Snack	Bedtime	Night	Notes
Blood Sugar									
Insulin Dose									
Grams Carb									
Activity									

Date:	Breakfast	Snack	Lunch	Snack	Dinner	Snack	Bedtime	Night	Notes
Blood Sugar									
Insulin Dose									
Grams Carb									
Activity									

Date:	Breakfast	Snack	Lunch	Snack	Dinner	Snack	Bedtime	Night	Notes
Blood Sugar									
Insulin Dose									
Grams Carb									
Activity									

Date:	Breakfast	Snack	Lunch	Snack	Dinner	Snack	Bedtime	Night	Notes
Blood Sugar									
Insulin Dose									
Grams Carb									
Activity									

Weekly Diabetes Record

Name: ______________________________

Date:	Breakfast	Snack	Lunch	Snack	Dinner	Snack	Bedtime	Night	Notes
Blood Sugar									
Insulin Dose									
Grams Carb									
Activity									

Date:	Breakfast	Snack	Lunch	Snack	Dinner	Snack	Bedtime	Night	Notes
Blood Sugar									
Insulin Dose									
Grams Carb									
Activity									

Date:	Breakfast	Snack	Lunch	Snack	Dinner	Snack	Bedtime	Night	Notes
Blood Sugar									
Insulin Dose									
Grams Carb									
Activity									

Date:	Breakfast	Snack	Lunch	Snack	Dinner	Snack	Bedtime	Night	Notes
Blood Sugar									
Insulin Dose									
Grams Carb									
Activity									

Date:	Breakfast	Snack	Lunch	Snack	Dinner	Snack	Bedtime	Night	Notes
Blood Sugar									
Insulin Dose									
Grams Carb									
Activity									

Date:	Breakfast	Snack	Lunch	Snack	Dinner	Snack	Bedtime	Night	Notes
Blood Sugar									
Insulin Dose									
Grams Carb									
Activity									

Date:	Breakfast	Snack	Lunch	Snack	Dinner	Snack	Bedtime	Night	Notes
Blood Sugar									
Insulin Dose									
Grams Carb									
Activity									

Weekly Diabetes Record

Name: ______________________________

Date:	Breakfast	Snack	Lunch	Snack	Dinner	Snack	Bedtime	Night	Notes
Blood Sugar									
Insulin Dose									
Grams Carb									
Activity									

Date:	Breakfast	Snack	Lunch	Snack	Dinner	Snack	Bedtime	Night	Notes
Blood Sugar									
Insulin Dose									
Grams Carb									
Activity									

Date:	Breakfast	Snack	Lunch	Snack	Dinner	Snack	Bedtime	Night	Notes
Blood Sugar									
Insulin Dose									
Grams Carb									
Activity									

Date:	Breakfast	Snack	Lunch	Snack	Dinner	Snack	Bedtime	Night	Notes
Blood Sugar									
Insulin Dose									
Grams Carb									
Activity									

Date:	Breakfast	Snack	Lunch	Snack	Dinner	Snack	Bedtime	Night	Notes
Blood Sugar									
Insulin Dose									
Grams Carb									
Activity									

Date:	Breakfast	Snack	Lunch	Snack	Dinner	Snack	Bedtime	Night	Notes
Blood Sugar									
Insulin Dose									
Grams Carb									
Activity									

Date:	Breakfast	Snack	Lunch	Snack	Dinner	Snack	Bedtime	Night	Notes
Blood Sugar									
Insulin Dose									
Grams Carb									
Activity									

Weekly Diabetes Record

Name: ______________________________

Date:	Breakfast	Snack	Lunch	Snack	Dinner	Snack	Bedtime	Night	Notes
Blood Sugar									
Insulin Dose									
Grams Carb									
Activity									

Date:	Breakfast	Snack	Lunch	Snack	Dinner	Snack	Bedtime	Night	Notes
Blood Sugar									
Insulin Dose									
Grams Carb									
Activity									

Date:	Breakfast	Snack	Lunch	Snack	Dinner	Snack	Bedtime	Night	Notes
Blood Sugar									
Insulin Dose									
Grams Carb									
Activity									

Date:	Breakfast	Snack	Lunch	Snack	Dinner	Snack	Bedtime	Night	Notes
Blood Sugar									
Insulin Dose									
Grams Carb									
Activity									

Date:	Breakfast	Snack	Lunch	Snack	Dinner	Snack	Bedtime	Night	Notes
Blood Sugar									
Insulin Dose									
Grams Carb									
Activity									

Date:	Breakfast	Snack	Lunch	Snack	Dinner	Snack	Bedtime	Night	Notes
Blood Sugar									
Insulin Dose									
Grams Carb									
Activity									

Date:	Breakfast	Snack	Lunch	Snack	Dinner	Snack	Bedtime	Night	Notes
Blood Sugar									
Insulin Dose									
Grams Carb									
Activity									

Weekly Diabetes Record

Name: ____

Date:	Breakfast	Snack	Lunch	Snack	Dinner	Snack	Bedtime	Night	Notes
Blood Sugar									
Insulin Dose									
Grams Carb									
Activity									

Date:	Breakfast	Snack	Lunch	Snack	Dinner	Snack	Bedtime	Night	Notes
Blood Sugar									
Insulin Dose									
Grams Carb									
Activity									

Date:	Breakfast	Snack	Lunch	Snack	Dinner	Snack	Bedtime	Night	Notes
Blood Sugar									
Insulin Dose									
Grams Carb									
Activity									

Date:	Breakfast	Snack	Lunch	Snack	Dinner	Snack	Bedtime	Night	Notes
Blood Sugar									
Insulin Dose									
Grams Carb									
Activity									

Date:	Breakfast	Snack	Lunch	Snack	Dinner	Snack	Bedtime	Night	Notes
Blood Sugar									
Insulin Dose									
Grams Carb									
Activity									

Date:	Breakfast	Snack	Lunch	Snack	Dinner	Snack	Bedtime	Night	Notes
Blood Sugar									
Insulin Dose									
Grams Carb									
Activity									

Date:	Breakfast	Snack	Lunch	Snack	Dinner	Snack	Bedtime	Night	Notes
Blood Sugar									
Insulin Dose									
Grams Carb									
Activity									

Weekly Diabetes Record

Name: ______________________________

Date:	Breakfast	Snack	Lunch	Snack	Dinner	Snack	Bedtime	Night	Notes
Blood Sugar									
Insulin Dose									
Grams Carb									
Activity									

Date:	Breakfast	Snack	Lunch	Snack	Dinner	Snack	Bedtime	Night	Notes
Blood Sugar									
Insulin Dose									
Grams Carb									
Activity									

Date:	Breakfast	Snack	Lunch	Snack	Dinner	Snack	Bedtime	Night	Notes
Blood Sugar									
Insulin Dose									
Grams Carb									
Activity									

Date:	Breakfast	Snack	Lunch	Snack	Dinner	Snack	Bedtime	Night	Notes
Blood Sugar									
Insulin Dose									
Grams Carb									
Activity									

Date:	Breakfast	Snack	Lunch	Snack	Dinner	Snack	Bedtime	Night	Notes
Blood Sugar									
Insulin Dose									
Grams Carb									
Activity									

Date:	Breakfast	Snack	Lunch	Snack	Dinner	Snack	Bedtime	Night	Notes
Blood Sugar									
Insulin Dose									
Grams Carb									
Activity									

Date:	Breakfast	Snack	Lunch	Snack	Dinner	Snack	Bedtime	Night	Notes
Blood Sugar									
Insulin Dose									
Grams Carb									
Activity									

Weekly Diabetes Record

Name: ______________________________

Date:	Breakfast	Snack	Lunch	Snack	Dinner	Snack	Bedtime	Night	Notes
Blood Sugar									
Insulin Dose									
Grams Carb									
Activity									

Date:	Breakfast	Snack	Lunch	Snack	Dinner	Snack	Bedtime	Night	Notes
Blood Sugar									
Insulin Dose									
Grams Carb									
Activity									

Date:	Breakfast	Snack	Lunch	Snack	Dinner	Snack	Bedtime	Night	Notes
Blood Sugar									
Insulin Dose									
Grams Carb									
Activity									

Date:	Breakfast	Snack	Lunch	Snack	Dinner	Snack	Bedtime	Night	Notes
Blood Sugar									
Insulin Dose									
Grams Carb									
Activity									

Date:	Breakfast	Snack	Lunch	Snack	Dinner	Snack	Bedtime	Night	Notes
Blood Sugar									
Insulin Dose									
Grams Carb									
Activity									

Date:	Breakfast	Snack	Lunch	Snack	Dinner	Snack	Bedtime	Night	Notes
Blood Sugar									
Insulin Dose									
Grams Carb									
Activity									

Date:	Breakfast	Snack	Lunch	Snack	Dinner	Snack	Bedtime	Night	Notes
Blood Sugar									
Insulin Dose									
Grams Carb									
Activity									

Weekly Diabetes Record

Name: ______________________________

Date:	Breakfast	Snack	Lunch	Snack	Dinner	Snack	Bedtime	Night	Notes
Blood Sugar									
Insulin Dose									
Grams Carb									
Activity									

Date:	Breakfast	Snack	Lunch	Snack	Dinner	Snack	Bedtime	Night	Notes
Blood Sugar									
Insulin Dose									
Grams Carb									
Activity									

Date:	Breakfast	Snack	Lunch	Snack	Dinner	Snack	Bedtime	Night	Notes
Blood Sugar									
Insulin Dose									
Grams Carb									
Activity									

Date:	Breakfast	Snack	Lunch	Snack	Dinner	Snack	Bedtime	Night	Notes
Blood Sugar									
Insulin Dose									
Grams Carb									
Activity									

Date:	Breakfast	Snack	Lunch	Snack	Dinner	Snack	Bedtime	Night	Notes
Blood Sugar									
Insulin Dose									
Grams Carb									
Activity									

Date:	Breakfast	Snack	Lunch	Snack	Dinner	Snack	Bedtime	Night	Notes
Blood Sugar									
Insulin Dose									
Grams Carb									
Activity									

Date:	Breakfast	Snack	Lunch	Snack	Dinner	Snack	Bedtime	Night	Notes
Blood Sugar									
Insulin Dose									
Grams Carb									
Activity									

Weekly Diabetes Record

Name: ______________________________

Date:	Breakfast	Snack	Lunch	Snack	Dinner	Snack	Bedtime	Night	Notes
Blood Sugar									
Insulin Dose									
Grams Carb									
Activity									

Date:	Breakfast	Snack	Lunch	Snack	Dinner	Snack	Bedtime	Night	Notes
Blood Sugar									
Insulin Dose									
Grams Carb									
Activity									

Date:	Breakfast	Snack	Lunch	Snack	Dinner	Snack	Bedtime	Night	Notes
Blood Sugar									
Insulin Dose									
Grams Carb									
Activity									

Date:	Breakfast	Snack	Lunch	Snack	Dinner	Snack	Bedtime	Night	Notes
Blood Sugar									
Insulin Dose									
Grams Carb									
Activity									

Date:	Breakfast	Snack	Lunch	Snack	Dinner	Snack	Bedtime	Night	Notes
Blood Sugar									
Insulin Dose									
Grams Carb									
Activity									

Date:	Breakfast	Snack	Lunch	Snack	Dinner	Snack	Bedtime	Night	Notes
Blood Sugar									
Insulin Dose									
Grams Carb									
Activity									

Date:	Breakfast	Snack	Lunch	Snack	Dinner	Snack	Bedtime	Night	Notes
Blood Sugar									
Insulin Dose									
Grams Carb									
Activity									

Weekly Diabetes Record

Name: ______________________________

Date:	Breakfast	Snack	Lunch	Snack	Dinner	Snack	Bedtime	Night	Notes
Blood Sugar									
Insulin Dose									
Grams Carb									
Activity									

Date:	Breakfast	Snack	Lunch	Snack	Dinner	Snack	Bedtime	Night	Notes
Blood Sugar									
Insulin Dose									
Grams Carb									
Activity									

Date:	Breakfast	Snack	Lunch	Snack	Dinner	Snack	Bedtime	Night	Notes
Blood Sugar									
Insulin Dose									
Grams Carb									
Activity									

Date:	Breakfast	Snack	Lunch	Snack	Dinner	Snack	Bedtime	Night	Notes
Blood Sugar									
Insulin Dose									
Grams Carb									
Activity									

Date:	Breakfast	Snack	Lunch	Snack	Dinner	Snack	Bedtime	Night	Notes
Blood Sugar									
Insulin Dose									
Grams Carb									
Activity									

Date:	Breakfast	Snack	Lunch	Snack	Dinner	Snack	Bedtime	Night	Notes
Blood Sugar									
Insulin Dose									
Grams Carb									
Activity									

Date:	Breakfast	Snack	Lunch	Snack	Dinner	Snack	Bedtime	Night	Notes
Blood Sugar									
Insulin Dose									
Grams Carb									
Activity									

Weekly Diabetes Record

Name: ____

Date:	Breakfast	Snack	Lunch	Snack	Dinner	Snack	Bedtime	Night	Notes
Blood Sugar									
Insulin Dose									
Grams Carb									
Activity									

Date:	Breakfast	Snack	Lunch	Snack	Dinner	Snack	Bedtime	Night	Notes
Blood Sugar									
Insulin Dose									
Grams Carb									
Activity									

Date:	Breakfast	Snack	Lunch	Snack	Dinner	Snack	Bedtime	Night	Notes
Blood Sugar									
Insulin Dose									
Grams Carb									
Activity									

Date:	Breakfast	Snack	Lunch	Snack	Dinner	Snack	Bedtime	Night	Notes
Blood Sugar									
Insulin Dose									
Grams Carb									
Activity									

Date:	Breakfast	Snack	Lunch	Snack	Dinner	Snack	Bedtime	Night	Notes
Blood Sugar									
Insulin Dose									
Grams Carb									
Activity									

Date:	Breakfast	Snack	Lunch	Snack	Dinner	Snack	Bedtime	Night	Notes
Blood Sugar									
Insulin Dose									
Grams Carb									
Activity									

Date:	Breakfast	Snack	Lunch	Snack	Dinner	Snack	Bedtime	Night	Notes
Blood Sugar									
Insulin Dose									
Grams Carb									
Activity									

Weekly Diabetes Record

Name: ______________________________

Date:	Breakfast	Snack	Lunch	Snack	Dinner	Snack	Bedtime	Night	Notes
Blood Sugar									
Insulin Dose									
Grams Carb									
Activity									

Date:	Breakfast	Snack	Lunch	Snack	Dinner	Snack	Bedtime	Night	Notes
Blood Sugar									
Insulin Dose									
Grams Carb									
Activity									

Date:	Breakfast	Snack	Lunch	Snack	Dinner	Snack	Bedtime	Night	Notes
Blood Sugar									
Insulin Dose									
Grams Carb									
Activity									

Date:	Breakfast	Snack	Lunch	Snack	Dinner	Snack	Bedtime	Night	Notes
Blood Sugar									
Insulin Dose									
Grams Carb									
Activity									

Date:	Breakfast	Snack	Lunch	Snack	Dinner	Snack	Bedtime	Night	Notes
Blood Sugar									
Insulin Dose									
Grams Carb									
Activity									

Date:	Breakfast	Snack	Lunch	Snack	Dinner	Snack	Bedtime	Night	Notes
Blood Sugar									
Insulin Dose									
Grams Carb									
Activity									

Date:	Breakfast	Snack	Lunch	Snack	Dinner	Snack	Bedtime	Night	Notes
Blood Sugar									
Insulin Dose									
Grams Carb									
Activity									

Weekly Diabetes Record

Name: ______________________________

Date:	Breakfast	Snack	Lunch	Snack	Dinner	Snack	Bedtime	Night	Notes
Blood Sugar									
Insulin Dose									
Grams Carb									
Activity									

Date:	Breakfast	Snack	Lunch	Snack	Dinner	Snack	Bedtime	Night	Notes
Blood Sugar									
Insulin Dose									
Grams Carb									
Activity									

Date:	Breakfast	Snack	Lunch	Snack	Dinner	Snack	Bedtime	Night	Notes
Blood Sugar									
Insulin Dose									
Grams Carb									
Activity									

Date:	Breakfast	Snack	Lunch	Snack	Dinner	Snack	Bedtime	Night	Notes
Blood Sugar									
Insulin Dose									
Grams Carb									
Activity									

Date:	Breakfast	Snack	Lunch	Snack	Dinner	Snack	Bedtime	Night	Notes
Blood Sugar									
Insulin Dose									
Grams Carb									
Activity									

Date:	Breakfast	Snack	Lunch	Snack	Dinner	Snack	Bedtime	Night	Notes
Blood Sugar									
Insulin Dose									
Grams Carb									
Activity									

Date:	Breakfast	Snack	Lunch	Snack	Dinner	Snack	Bedtime	Night	Notes
Blood Sugar									
Insulin Dose									
Grams Carb									
Activity									

Weekly Diabetes Record

Name: ______________________________

Date:	Breakfast	Snack	Lunch	Snack	Dinner	Snack	Bedtime	Night	Notes
Blood Sugar									
Insulin Dose									
Grams Carb									
Activity									

Date:	Breakfast	Snack	Lunch	Snack	Dinner	Snack	Bedtime	Night	Notes
Blood Sugar									
Insulin Dose									
Grams Carb									
Activity									

Date:	Breakfast	Snack	Lunch	Snack	Dinner	Snack	Bedtime	Night	Notes
Blood Sugar									
Insulin Dose									
Grams Carb									
Activity									

Date:	Breakfast	Snack	Lunch	Snack	Dinner	Snack	Bedtime	Night	Notes
Blood Sugar									
Insulin Dose									
Grams Carb									
Activity									

Date:	Breakfast	Snack	Lunch	Snack	Dinner	Snack	Bedtime	Night	Notes
Blood Sugar									
Insulin Dose									
Grams Carb									
Activity									

Date:	Breakfast	Snack	Lunch	Snack	Dinner	Snack	Bedtime	Night	Notes
Blood Sugar									
Insulin Dose									
Grams Carb									
Activity									

Date:	Breakfast	Snack	Lunch	Snack	Dinner	Snack	Bedtime	Night	Notes
Blood Sugar									
Insulin Dose									
Grams Carb									
Activity									

Weekly Diabetes Record

Name: ______________________________

Date:	Breakfast	Snack	Lunch	Snack	Dinner	Snack	Bedtime	Night	Notes
Blood Sugar									
Insulin Dose									
Grams Carb									
Activity									

Date:	Breakfast	Snack	Lunch	Snack	Dinner	Snack	Bedtime	Night	Notes
Blood Sugar									
Insulin Dose									
Grams Carb									
Activity									

Date:	Breakfast	Snack	Lunch	Snack	Dinner	Snack	Bedtime	Night	Notes
Blood Sugar									
Insulin Dose									
Grams Carb									
Activity									

Date:	Breakfast	Snack	Lunch	Snack	Dinner	Snack	Bedtime	Night	Notes
Blood Sugar									
Insulin Dose									
Grams Carb									
Activity									

Date:	Breakfast	Snack	Lunch	Snack	Dinner	Snack	Bedtime	Night	Notes
Blood Sugar									
Insulin Dose									
Grams Carb									
Activity									

Date:	Breakfast	Snack	Lunch	Snack	Dinner	Snack	Bedtime	Night	Notes
Blood Sugar									
Insulin Dose									
Grams Carb									
Activity									

Date:	Breakfast	Snack	Lunch	Snack	Dinner	Snack	Bedtime	Night	Notes
Blood Sugar									
Insulin Dose									
Grams Carb									
Activity									

Weekly Diabetes Record

Name: ____

Date:	Breakfast	Snack	Lunch	Snack	Dinner	Snack	Bedtime	Night	Notes
Blood Sugar									
Insulin Dose									
Grams Carb									
Activity									

Date:	Breakfast	Snack	Lunch	Snack	Dinner	Snack	Bedtime	Night	Notes
Blood Sugar									
Insulin Dose									
Grams Carb									
Activity									

Date:	Breakfast	Snack	Lunch	Snack	Dinner	Snack	Bedtime	Night	Notes
Blood Sugar									
Insulin Dose									
Grams Carb									
Activity									

Date:	Breakfast	Snack	Lunch	Snack	Dinner	Snack	Bedtime	Night	Notes
Blood Sugar									
Insulin Dose									
Grams Carb									
Activity									

Date:	Breakfast	Snack	Lunch	Snack	Dinner	Snack	Bedtime	Night	Notes
Blood Sugar									
Insulin Dose									
Grams Carb									
Activity									

Date:	Breakfast	Snack	Lunch	Snack	Dinner	Snack	Bedtime	Night	Notes
Blood Sugar									
Insulin Dose									
Grams Carb									
Activity									

Date:	Breakfast	Snack	Lunch	Snack	Dinner	Snack	Bedtime	Night	Notes
Blood Sugar									
Insulin Dose									
Grams Carb									
Activity									

Weekly Diabetes Record

Name: ____

Date:	Breakfast	Snack	Lunch	Snack	Dinner	Snack	Bedtime	Night	Notes
Blood Sugar									
Insulin Dose									
Grams Carb									
Activity									

Date:	Breakfast	Snack	Lunch	Snack	Dinner	Snack	Bedtime	Night	Notes
Blood Sugar									
Insulin Dose									
Grams Carb									
Activity									

Date:	Breakfast	Snack	Lunch	Snack	Dinner	Snack	Bedtime	Night	Notes
Blood Sugar									
Insulin Dose									
Grams Carb									
Activity									

Date:	Breakfast	Snack	Lunch	Snack	Dinner	Snack	Bedtime	Night	Notes
Blood Sugar									
Insulin Dose									
Grams Carb									
Activity									

Date:	Breakfast	Snack	Lunch	Snack	Dinner	Snack	Bedtime	Night	Notes
Blood Sugar									
Insulin Dose									
Grams Carb									
Activity									

Date:	Breakfast	Snack	Lunch	Snack	Dinner	Snack	Bedtime	Night	Notes
Blood Sugar									
Insulin Dose									
Grams Carb									
Activity									

Date:	Breakfast	Snack	Lunch	Snack	Dinner	Snack	Bedtime	Night	Notes
Blood Sugar									
Insulin Dose									
Grams Carb									
Activity									

Weekly Diabetes Record

Name: ______________________________

Date:	Breakfast	Snack	Lunch	Snack	Dinner	Snack	Bedtime	Night	Notes
Blood Sugar									
Insulin Dose									
Grams Carb									
Activity									

Date:	Breakfast	Snack	Lunch	Snack	Dinner	Snack	Bedtime	Night	Notes
Blood Sugar									
Insulin Dose									
Grams Carb									
Activity									

Date:	Breakfast	Snack	Lunch	Snack	Dinner	Snack	Bedtime	Night	Notes
Blood Sugar									
Insulin Dose									
Grams Carb									
Activity									

Date:	Breakfast	Snack	Lunch	Snack	Dinner	Snack	Bedtime	Night	Notes
Blood Sugar									
Insulin Dose									
Grams Carb									
Activity									

Date:	Breakfast	Snack	Lunch	Snack	Dinner	Snack	Bedtime	Night	Notes
Blood Sugar									
Insulin Dose									
Grams Carb									
Activity									

Date:	Breakfast	Snack	Lunch	Snack	Dinner	Snack	Bedtime	Night	Notes
Blood Sugar									
Insulin Dose									
Grams Carb									
Activity									

Date:	Breakfast	Snack	Lunch	Snack	Dinner	Snack	Bedtime	Night	Notes
Blood Sugar									
Insulin Dose									
Grams Carb									
Activity									

Weekly Diabetes Record

Name: ______________________________

Date:	Breakfast	Snack	Lunch	Snack	Dinner	Snack	Bedtime	Night	Notes
Blood Sugar									
Insulin Dose									
Grams Carb									
Activity									

Date:	Breakfast	Snack	Lunch	Snack	Dinner	Snack	Bedtime	Night	Notes
Blood Sugar									
Insulin Dose									
Grams Carb									
Activity									

Date:	Breakfast	Snack	Lunch	Snack	Dinner	Snack	Bedtime	Night	Notes
Blood Sugar									
Insulin Dose									
Grams Carb									
Activity									

Date:	Breakfast	Snack	Lunch	Snack	Dinner	Snack	Bedtime	Night	Notes
Blood Sugar									
Insulin Dose									
Grams Carb									
Activity									

Date:	Breakfast	Snack	Lunch	Snack	Dinner	Snack	Bedtime	Night	Notes
Blood Sugar									
Insulin Dose									
Grams Carb									
Activity									

Date:	Breakfast	Snack	Lunch	Snack	Dinner	Snack	Bedtime	Night	Notes
Blood Sugar									
Insulin Dose									
Grams Carb									
Activity									

Date:	Breakfast	Snack	Lunch	Snack	Dinner	Snack	Bedtime	Night	Notes
Blood Sugar									
Insulin Dose									
Grams Carb									
Activity									

Weekly Diabetes Record

Name: ______________________________

Date:	Breakfast	Snack	Lunch	Snack	Dinner	Snack	Bedtime	Night	Notes
Blood Sugar									
Insulin Dose									
Grams Carb									
Activity									

Date:	Breakfast	Snack	Lunch	Snack	Dinner	Snack	Bedtime	Night	Notes
Blood Sugar									
Insulin Dose									
Grams Carb									
Activity									

Date:	Breakfast	Snack	Lunch	Snack	Dinner	Snack	Bedtime	Night	Notes
Blood Sugar									
Insulin Dose									
Grams Carb									
Activity									

Date:	Breakfast	Snack	Lunch	Snack	Dinner	Snack	Bedtime	Night	Notes
Blood Sugar									
Insulin Dose									
Grams Carb									
Activity									

Date:	Breakfast	Snack	Lunch	Snack	Dinner	Snack	Bedtime	Night	Notes
Blood Sugar									
Insulin Dose									
Grams Carb									
Activity									

Date:	Breakfast	Snack	Lunch	Snack	Dinner	Snack	Bedtime	Night	Notes
Blood Sugar									
Insulin Dose									
Grams Carb									
Activity									

Date:	Breakfast	Snack	Lunch	Snack	Dinner	Snack	Bedtime	Night	Notes
Blood Sugar									
Insulin Dose									
Grams Carb									
Activity									

Weekly Diabetes Record

Name: ______________________________

Date:	Breakfast	Snack	Lunch	Snack	Dinner	Snack	Bedtime	Night	Notes
Blood Sugar									
Insulin Dose									
Grams Carb									
Activity									

Date:	Breakfast	Snack	Lunch	Snack	Dinner	Snack	Bedtime	Night	Notes
Blood Sugar									
Insulin Dose									
Grams Carb									
Activity									

Date:	Breakfast	Snack	Lunch	Snack	Dinner	Snack	Bedtime	Night	Notes
Blood Sugar									
Insulin Dose									
Grams Carb									
Activity									

Date:	Breakfast	Snack	Lunch	Snack	Dinner	Snack	Bedtime	Night	Notes
Blood Sugar									
Insulin Dose									
Grams Carb									
Activity									

Date:	Breakfast	Snack	Lunch	Snack	Dinner	Snack	Bedtime	Night	Notes
Blood Sugar									
Insulin Dose									
Grams Carb									
Activity									

Date:	Breakfast	Snack	Lunch	Snack	Dinner	Snack	Bedtime	Night	Notes
Blood Sugar									
Insulin Dose									
Grams Carb									
Activity									

Date:	Breakfast	Snack	Lunch	Snack	Dinner	Snack	Bedtime	Night	Notes
Blood Sugar									
Insulin Dose									
Grams Carb									
Activity									

Weekly Diabetes Record

Name: ______________________________

Date:	Breakfast	Snack	Lunch	Snack	Dinner	Snack	Bedtime	Night	Notes
Blood Sugar									
Insulin Dose									
Grams Carb									
Activity									

Date:	Breakfast	Snack	Lunch	Snack	Dinner	Snack	Bedtime	Night	Notes
Blood Sugar									
Insulin Dose									
Grams Carb									
Activity									

Date:	Breakfast	Snack	Lunch	Snack	Dinner	Snack	Bedtime	Night	Notes
Blood Sugar									
Insulin Dose									
Grams Carb									
Activity									

Date:	Breakfast	Snack	Lunch	Snack	Dinner	Snack	Bedtime	Night	Notes
Blood Sugar									
Insulin Dose									
Grams Carb									
Activity									

Date:	Breakfast	Snack	Lunch	Snack	Dinner	Snack	Bedtime	Night	Notes
Blood Sugar									
Insulin Dose									
Grams Carb									
Activity									

Date:	Breakfast	Snack	Lunch	Snack	Dinner	Snack	Bedtime	Night	Notes
Blood Sugar									
Insulin Dose									
Grams Carb									
Activity									

Date:	Breakfast	Snack	Lunch	Snack	Dinner	Snack	Bedtime	Night	Notes
Blood Sugar									
Insulin Dose									
Grams Carb									
Activity									

Weekly Diabetes Record

Name: ______________________________

Date:	Breakfast	Snack	Lunch	Snack	Dinner	Snack	Bedtime	Night	Notes
Blood Sugar									
Insulin Dose									
Grams Carb									
Activity									

Date:	Breakfast	Snack	Lunch	Snack	Dinner	Snack	Bedtime	Night	Notes
Blood Sugar									
Insulin Dose									
Grams Carb									
Activity									

Date:	Breakfast	Snack	Lunch	Snack	Dinner	Snack	Bedtime	Night	Notes
Blood Sugar									
Insulin Dose									
Grams Carb									
Activity									

Date:	Breakfast	Snack	Lunch	Snack	Dinner	Snack	Bedtime	Night	Notes
Blood Sugar									
Insulin Dose									
Grams Carb									
Activity									

Date:	Breakfast	Snack	Lunch	Snack	Dinner	Snack	Bedtime	Night	Notes
Blood Sugar									
Insulin Dose									
Grams Carb									
Activity									

Date:	Breakfast	Snack	Lunch	Snack	Dinner	Snack	Bedtime	Night	Notes
Blood Sugar									
Insulin Dose									
Grams Carb									
Activity									

Date:	Breakfast	Snack	Lunch	Snack	Dinner	Snack	Bedtime	Night	Notes
Blood Sugar									
Insulin Dose									
Grams Carb									
Activity									

Weekly Diabetes Record

Name: ______________________________

Date:	Breakfast	Snack	Lunch	Snack	Dinner	Snack	Bedtime	Night	Notes
Blood Sugar									
Insulin Dose									
Grams Carb									
Activity									

Date:	Breakfast	Snack	Lunch	Snack	Dinner	Snack	Bedtime	Night	Notes
Blood Sugar									
Insulin Dose									
Grams Carb									
Activity									

Date:	Breakfast	Snack	Lunch	Snack	Dinner	Snack	Bedtime	Night	Notes
Blood Sugar									
Insulin Dose									
Grams Carb									
Activity									

Date:	Breakfast	Snack	Lunch	Snack	Dinner	Snack	Bedtime	Night	Notes
Blood Sugar									
Insulin Dose									
Grams Carb									
Activity									

Date:	Breakfast	Snack	Lunch	Snack	Dinner	Snack	Bedtime	Night	Notes
Blood Sugar									
Insulin Dose									
Grams Carb									
Activity									

Date:	Breakfast	Snack	Lunch	Snack	Dinner	Snack	Bedtime	Night	Notes
Blood Sugar									
Insulin Dose									
Grams Carb									
Activity									

Date:	Breakfast	Snack	Lunch	Snack	Dinner	Snack	Bedtime	Night	Notes
Blood Sugar									
Insulin Dose									
Grams Carb									
Activity									

Weekly Diabetes Record

Name: ______________________________

Date:	Breakfast	Snack	Lunch	Snack	Dinner	Snack	Bedtime	Night	Notes
Blood Sugar									
Insulin Dose									
Grams Carb									
Activity									

Date:	Breakfast	Snack	Lunch	Snack	Dinner	Snack	Bedtime	Night	Notes
Blood Sugar									
Insulin Dose									
Grams Carb									
Activity									

Date:	Breakfast	Snack	Lunch	Snack	Dinner	Snack	Bedtime	Night	Notes
Blood Sugar									
Insulin Dose									
Grams Carb									
Activity									

Date:	Breakfast	Snack	Lunch	Snack	Dinner	Snack	Bedtime	Night	Notes
Blood Sugar									
Insulin Dose									
Grams Carb									
Activity									

Date:	Breakfast	Snack	Lunch	Snack	Dinner	Snack	Bedtime	Night	Notes
Blood Sugar									
Insulin Dose									
Grams Carb									
Activity									

Date:	Breakfast	Snack	Lunch	Snack	Dinner	Snack	Bedtime	Night	Notes
Blood Sugar									
Insulin Dose									
Grams Carb									
Activity									

Date:	Breakfast	Snack	Lunch	Snack	Dinner	Snack	Bedtime	Night	Notes
Blood Sugar									
Insulin Dose									
Grams Carb									
Activity									

Weekly Diabetes Record

Name: ______________________________

Date:	Breakfast	Snack	Lunch	Snack	Dinner	Snack	Bedtime	Night	Notes
Blood Sugar									
Insulin Dose									
Grams Carb									
Activity									

Date:	Breakfast	Snack	Lunch	Snack	Dinner	Snack	Bedtime	Night	Notes
Blood Sugar									
Insulin Dose									
Grams Carb									
Activity									

Date:	Breakfast	Snack	Lunch	Snack	Dinner	Snack	Bedtime	Night	Notes
Blood Sugar									
Insulin Dose									
Grams Carb									
Activity									

Date:	Breakfast	Snack	Lunch	Snack	Dinner	Snack	Bedtime	Night	Notes
Blood Sugar									
Insulin Dose									
Grams Carb									
Activity									

Date:	Breakfast	Snack	Lunch	Snack	Dinner	Snack	Bedtime	Night	Notes
Blood Sugar									
Insulin Dose									
Grams Carb									
Activity									

Date:	Breakfast	Snack	Lunch	Snack	Dinner	Snack	Bedtime	Night	Notes
Blood Sugar									
Insulin Dose									
Grams Carb									
Activity									

Date:	Breakfast	Snack	Lunch	Snack	Dinner	Snack	Bedtime	Night	Notes
Blood Sugar									
Insulin Dose									
Grams Carb									
Activity									

Weekly Diabetes Record

Name: ______________________________

Date:	Breakfast	Snack	Lunch	Snack	Dinner	Snack	Bedtime	Night	Notes
Blood Sugar									
Insulin Dose									
Grams Carb									
Activity									

Date:	Breakfast	Snack	Lunch	Snack	Dinner	Snack	Bedtime	Night	Notes
Blood Sugar									
Insulin Dose									
Grams Carb									
Activity									

Date:	Breakfast	Snack	Lunch	Snack	Dinner	Snack	Bedtime	Night	Notes
Blood Sugar									
Insulin Dose									
Grams Carb									
Activity									

Date:	Breakfast	Snack	Lunch	Snack	Dinner	Snack	Bedtime	Night	Notes
Blood Sugar									
Insulin Dose									
Grams Carb									
Activity									

Date:	Breakfast	Snack	Lunch	Snack	Dinner	Snack	Bedtime	Night	Notes
Blood Sugar									
Insulin Dose									
Grams Carb									
Activity									

Date:	Breakfast	Snack	Lunch	Snack	Dinner	Snack	Bedtime	Night	Notes
Blood Sugar									
Insulin Dose									
Grams Carb									
Activity									

Date:	Breakfast	Snack	Lunch	Snack	Dinner	Snack	Bedtime	Night	Notes
Blood Sugar									
Insulin Dose									
Grams Carb									
Activity									

Weekly Diabetes Record

Name: ______________________________

Date:	Breakfast	Snack	Lunch	Snack	Dinner	Snack	Bedtime	Night	Notes
Blood Sugar									
Insulin Dose									
Grams Carb									
Activity									

Date:	Breakfast	Snack	Lunch	Snack	Dinner	Snack	Bedtime	Night	Notes
Blood Sugar									
Insulin Dose									
Grams Carb									
Activity									

Date:	Breakfast	Snack	Lunch	Snack	Dinner	Snack	Bedtime	Night	Notes
Blood Sugar									
Insulin Dose									
Grams Carb									
Activity									

Date:	Breakfast	Snack	Lunch	Snack	Dinner	Snack	Bedtime	Night	Notes
Blood Sugar									
Insulin Dose									
Grams Carb									
Activity									

Date:	Breakfast	Snack	Lunch	Snack	Dinner	Snack	Bedtime	Night	Notes
Blood Sugar									
Insulin Dose									
Grams Carb									
Activity									

Date:	Breakfast	Snack	Lunch	Snack	Dinner	Snack	Bedtime	Night	Notes
Blood Sugar									
Insulin Dose									
Grams Carb									
Activity									

Date:	Breakfast	Snack	Lunch	Snack	Dinner	Snack	Bedtime	Night	Notes
Blood Sugar									
Insulin Dose									
Grams Carb									
Activity									

Weekly Diabetes Record

Name: ____________________

Date:	Breakfast	Snack	Lunch	Snack	Dinner	Snack	Bedtime	Night	Notes
Blood Sugar									
Insulin Dose									
Grams Carb									
Activity									

Date:	Breakfast	Snack	Lunch	Snack	Dinner	Snack	Bedtime	Night	Notes
Blood Sugar									
Insulin Dose									
Grams Carb									
Activity									

Date:	Breakfast	Snack	Lunch	Snack	Dinner	Snack	Bedtime	Night	Notes
Blood Sugar									
Insulin Dose									
Grams Carb									
Activity									

Date:	Breakfast	Snack	Lunch	Snack	Dinner	Snack	Bedtime	Night	Notes
Blood Sugar									
Insulin Dose									
Grams Carb									
Activity									

Date:	Breakfast	Snack	Lunch	Snack	Dinner	Snack	Bedtime	Night	Notes
Blood Sugar									
Insulin Dose									
Grams Carb									
Activity									

Date:	Breakfast	Snack	Lunch	Snack	Dinner	Snack	Bedtime	Night	Notes
Blood Sugar									
Insulin Dose									
Grams Carb									
Activity									

Date:	Breakfast	Snack	Lunch	Snack	Dinner	Snack	Bedtime	Night	Notes
Blood Sugar									
Insulin Dose									
Grams Carb									
Activity									

Weekly Diabetes Record

Name: ________________________________

Date:	Breakfast	Snack	Lunch	Snack	Dinner	Snack	Bedtime	Night	Notes
Blood Sugar									
Insulin Dose									
Grams Carb									
Activity									

Date:	Breakfast	Snack	Lunch	Snack	Dinner	Snack	Bedtime	Night	Notes
Blood Sugar									
Insulin Dose									
Grams Carb									
Activity									

Date:	Breakfast	Snack	Lunch	Snack	Dinner	Snack	Bedtime	Night	Notes
Blood Sugar									
Insulin Dose									
Grams Carb									
Activity									

Date:	Breakfast	Snack	Lunch	Snack	Dinner	Snack	Bedtime	Night	Notes
Blood Sugar									
Insulin Dose									
Grams Carb									
Activity									

Date:	Breakfast	Snack	Lunch	Snack	Dinner	Snack	Bedtime	Night	Notes
Blood Sugar									
Insulin Dose									
Grams Carb									
Activity									

Date:	Breakfast	Snack	Lunch	Snack	Dinner	Snack	Bedtime	Night	Notes
Blood Sugar									
Insulin Dose									
Grams Carb									
Activity									

Date:	Breakfast	Snack	Lunch	Snack	Dinner	Snack	Bedtime	Night	Notes
Blood Sugar									
Insulin Dose									
Grams Carb									
Activity									

Weekly Diabetes Record

Name: ______________________________

Date:	Breakfast	Snack	Lunch	Snack	Dinner	Snack	Bedtime	Night	Notes
Blood Sugar									
Insulin Dose									
Grams Carb									
Activity									

Date:	Breakfast	Snack	Lunch	Snack	Dinner	Snack	Bedtime	Night	Notes
Blood Sugar									
Insulin Dose									
Grams Carb									
Activity									

Date:	Breakfast	Snack	Lunch	Snack	Dinner	Snack	Bedtime	Night	Notes
Blood Sugar									
Insulin Dose									
Grams Carb									
Activity									

Date:	Breakfast	Snack	Lunch	Snack	Dinner	Snack	Bedtime	Night	Notes
Blood Sugar									
Insulin Dose									
Grams Carb									
Activity									

Date:	Breakfast	Snack	Lunch	Snack	Dinner	Snack	Bedtime	Night	Notes
Blood Sugar									
Insulin Dose									
Grams Carb									
Activity									

Date:	Breakfast	Snack	Lunch	Snack	Dinner	Snack	Bedtime	Night	Notes
Blood Sugar									
Insulin Dose									
Grams Carb									
Activity									

Date:	Breakfast	Snack	Lunch	Snack	Dinner	Snack	Bedtime	Night	Notes
Blood Sugar									
Insulin Dose									
Grams Carb									
Activity									

Weekly Diabetes Record

Name: ____

Date:	Breakfast	Snack	Lunch	Snack	Dinner	Snack	Bedtime	Night	Notes
Blood Sugar									
Insulin Dose									
Grams Carb									
Activity									

Date:	Breakfast	Snack	Lunch	Snack	Dinner	Snack	Bedtime	Night	Notes
Blood Sugar									
Insulin Dose									
Grams Carb									
Activity									

Date:	Breakfast	Snack	Lunch	Snack	Dinner	Snack	Bedtime	Night	Notes
Blood Sugar									
Insulin Dose									
Grams Carb									
Activity									

Date:	Breakfast	Snack	Lunch	Snack	Dinner	Snack	Bedtime	Night	Notes
Blood Sugar									
Insulin Dose									
Grams Carb									
Activity									

Date:	Breakfast	Snack	Lunch	Snack	Dinner	Snack	Bedtime	Night	Notes
Blood Sugar									
Insulin Dose									
Grams Carb									
Activity									

Date:	Breakfast	Snack	Lunch	Snack	Dinner	Snack	Bedtime	Night	Notes
Blood Sugar									
Insulin Dose									
Grams Carb									
Activity									

Date:	Breakfast	Snack	Lunch	Snack	Dinner	Snack	Bedtime	Night	Notes
Blood Sugar									
Insulin Dose									
Grams Carb									
Activity									

Weekly Diabetes Record

Name: ________________________________

Date:	Breakfast	Snack	Lunch	Snack	Dinner	Snack	Bedtime	Night	Notes
Blood Sugar									
Insulin Dose									
Grams Carb									
Activity									

Date:	Breakfast	Snack	Lunch	Snack	Dinner	Snack	Bedtime	Night	Notes
Blood Sugar									
Insulin Dose									
Grams Carb									
Activity									

Date:	Breakfast	Snack	Lunch	Snack	Dinner	Snack	Bedtime	Night	Notes
Blood Sugar									
Insulin Dose									
Grams Carb									
Activity									

Date:	Breakfast	Snack	Lunch	Snack	Dinner	Snack	Bedtime	Night	Notes
Blood Sugar									
Insulin Dose									
Grams Carb									
Activity									

Date:	Breakfast	Snack	Lunch	Snack	Dinner	Snack	Bedtime	Night	Notes
Blood Sugar									
Insulin Dose									
Grams Carb									
Activity									

Date:	Breakfast	Snack	Lunch	Snack	Dinner	Snack	Bedtime	Night	Notes
Blood Sugar									
Insulin Dose									
Grams Carb									
Activity									

Date:	Breakfast	Snack	Lunch	Snack	Dinner	Snack	Bedtime	Night	Notes
Blood Sugar									
Insulin Dose									
Grams Carb									
Activity									

Weekly Diabetes Record

Name: ______________________________

Date:	Breakfast	Snack	Lunch	Snack	Dinner	Snack	Bedtime	Night	Notes
Blood Sugar									
Insulin Dose									
Grams Carb									
Activity									

Date:	Breakfast	Snack	Lunch	Snack	Dinner	Snack	Bedtime	Night	Notes
Blood Sugar									
Insulin Dose									
Grams Carb									
Activity									

Date:	Breakfast	Snack	Lunch	Snack	Dinner	Snack	Bedtime	Night	Notes
Blood Sugar									
Insulin Dose									
Grams Carb									
Activity									

Date:	Breakfast	Snack	Lunch	Snack	Dinner	Snack	Bedtime	Night	Notes
Blood Sugar									
Insulin Dose									
Grams Carb									
Activity									

Date:	Breakfast	Snack	Lunch	Snack	Dinner	Snack	Bedtime	Night	Notes
Blood Sugar									
Insulin Dose									
Grams Carb									
Activity									

Date:	Breakfast	Snack	Lunch	Snack	Dinner	Snack	Bedtime	Night	Notes
Blood Sugar									
Insulin Dose									
Grams Carb									
Activity									

Date:	Breakfast	Snack	Lunch	Snack	Dinner	Snack	Bedtime	Night	Notes
Blood Sugar									
Insulin Dose									
Grams Carb									
Activity									

Weekly Diabetes Record

Name: ______________________________

Date:	Breakfast	Snack	Lunch	Snack	Dinner	Snack	Bedtime	Night	Notes
Blood Sugar									
Insulin Dose									
Grams Carb									
Activity									

Date:	Breakfast	Snack	Lunch	Snack	Dinner	Snack	Bedtime	Night	Notes
Blood Sugar									
Insulin Dose									
Grams Carb									
Activity									

Date:	Breakfast	Snack	Lunch	Snack	Dinner	Snack	Bedtime	Night	Notes
Blood Sugar									
Insulin Dose									
Grams Carb									
Activity									

Date:	Breakfast	Snack	Lunch	Snack	Dinner	Snack	Bedtime	Night	Notes
Blood Sugar									
Insulin Dose									
Grams Carb									
Activity									

Date:	Breakfast	Snack	Lunch	Snack	Dinner	Snack	Bedtime	Night	Notes
Blood Sugar									
Insulin Dose									
Grams Carb									
Activity									

Date:	Breakfast	Snack	Lunch	Snack	Dinner	Snack	Bedtime	Night	Notes
Blood Sugar									
Insulin Dose									
Grams Carb									
Activity									

Date:	Breakfast	Snack	Lunch	Snack	Dinner	Snack	Bedtime	Night	Notes
Blood Sugar									
Insulin Dose									
Grams Carb									
Activity									

Weekly Diabetes Record

Name: ______________________________

Date:	Breakfast	Snack	Lunch	Snack	Dinner	Snack	Bedtime	Night	Notes
Blood Sugar									
Insulin Dose									
Grams Carb									
Activity									

Date:	Breakfast	Snack	Lunch	Snack	Dinner	Snack	Bedtime	Night	Notes
Blood Sugar									
Insulin Dose									
Grams Carb									
Activity									

Date:	Breakfast	Snack	Lunch	Snack	Dinner	Snack	Bedtime	Night	Notes
Blood Sugar									
Insulin Dose									
Grams Carb									
Activity									

Date:	Breakfast	Snack	Lunch	Snack	Dinner	Snack	Bedtime	Night	Notes
Blood Sugar									
Insulin Dose									
Grams Carb									
Activity									

Date:	Breakfast	Snack	Lunch	Snack	Dinner	Snack	Bedtime	Night	Notes
Blood Sugar									
Insulin Dose									
Grams Carb									
Activity									

Date:	Breakfast	Snack	Lunch	Snack	Dinner	Snack	Bedtime	Night	Notes
Blood Sugar									
Insulin Dose									
Grams Carb									
Activity									

Date:	Breakfast	Snack	Lunch	Snack	Dinner	Snack	Bedtime	Night	Notes
Blood Sugar									
Insulin Dose									
Grams Carb									
Activity									

Weekly Diabetes Record

Name: ____

Date:	Breakfast	Snack	Lunch	Snack	Dinner	Snack	Bedtime	Night	Notes
Blood Sugar									
Insulin Dose									
Grams Carb									
Activity									

Date:	Breakfast	Snack	Lunch	Snack	Dinner	Snack	Bedtime	Night	Notes
Blood Sugar									
Insulin Dose									
Grams Carb									
Activity									

Date:	Breakfast	Snack	Lunch	Snack	Dinner	Snack	Bedtime	Night	Notes
Blood Sugar									
Insulin Dose									
Grams Carb									
Activity									

Date:	Breakfast	Snack	Lunch	Snack	Dinner	Snack	Bedtime	Night	Notes
Blood Sugar									
Insulin Dose									
Grams Carb									
Activity									

Date:	Breakfast	Snack	Lunch	Snack	Dinner	Snack	Bedtime	Night	Notes
Blood Sugar									
Insulin Dose									
Grams Carb									
Activity									

Date:	Breakfast	Snack	Lunch	Snack	Dinner	Snack	Bedtime	Night	Notes
Blood Sugar									
Insulin Dose									
Grams Carb									
Activity									

Date:	Breakfast	Snack	Lunch	Snack	Dinner	Snack	Bedtime	Night	Notes
Blood Sugar									
Insulin Dose									
Grams Carb									
Activity									

Weekly Diabetes Record

Name: ______________________________

Date:	Breakfast	Snack	Lunch	Snack	Dinner	Snack	Bedtime	Night	Notes
Blood Sugar									
Insulin Dose									
Grams Carb									
Activity									

Date:	Breakfast	Snack	Lunch	Snack	Dinner	Snack	Bedtime	Night	Notes
Blood Sugar									
Insulin Dose									
Grams Carb									
Activity									

Date:	Breakfast	Snack	Lunch	Snack	Dinner	Snack	Bedtime	Night	Notes
Blood Sugar									
Insulin Dose									
Grams Carb									
Activity									

Date:	Breakfast	Snack	Lunch	Snack	Dinner	Snack	Bedtime	Night	Notes
Blood Sugar									
Insulin Dose									
Grams Carb									
Activity									

Date:	Breakfast	Snack	Lunch	Snack	Dinner	Snack	Bedtime	Night	Notes
Blood Sugar									
Insulin Dose									
Grams Carb									
Activity									

Date:	Breakfast	Snack	Lunch	Snack	Dinner	Snack	Bedtime	Night	Notes
Blood Sugar									
Insulin Dose									
Grams Carb									
Activity									

Date:	Breakfast	Snack	Lunch	Snack	Dinner	Snack	Bedtime	Night	Notes
Blood Sugar									
Insulin Dose									
Grams Carb									
Activity									

Weekly Diabetes Record

Name: ______________________________

Date:	Breakfast	Snack	Lunch	Snack	Dinner	Snack	Bedtime	Night	Notes
Blood Sugar									
Insulin Dose									
Grams Carb									
Activity									

Date:	Breakfast	Snack	Lunch	Snack	Dinner	Snack	Bedtime	Night	Notes
Blood Sugar									
Insulin Dose									
Grams Carb									
Activity									

Date:	Breakfast	Snack	Lunch	Snack	Dinner	Snack	Bedtime	Night	Notes
Blood Sugar									
Insulin Dose									
Grams Carb									
Activity									

Date:	Breakfast	Snack	Lunch	Snack	Dinner	Snack	Bedtime	Night	Notes
Blood Sugar									
Insulin Dose									
Grams Carb									
Activity									

Date:	Breakfast	Snack	Lunch	Snack	Dinner	Snack	Bedtime	Night	Notes
Blood Sugar									
Insulin Dose									
Grams Carb									
Activity									

Date:	Breakfast	Snack	Lunch	Snack	Dinner	Snack	Bedtime	Night	Notes
Blood Sugar									
Insulin Dose									
Grams Carb									
Activity									

Date:	Breakfast	Snack	Lunch	Snack	Dinner	Snack	Bedtime	Night	Notes
Blood Sugar									
Insulin Dose									
Grams Carb									
Activity									

Weekly Diabetes Record

Name: ______________________________

Date:	Breakfast	Snack	Lunch	Snack	Dinner	Snack	Bedtime	Night	Notes
Blood Sugar									
Insulin Dose									
Grams Carb									
Activity									

Date:	Breakfast	Snack	Lunch	Snack	Dinner	Snack	Bedtime	Night	Notes
Blood Sugar									
Insulin Dose									
Grams Carb									
Activity									

Date:	Breakfast	Snack	Lunch	Snack	Dinner	Snack	Bedtime	Night	Notes
Blood Sugar									
Insulin Dose									
Grams Carb									
Activity									

Date:	Breakfast	Snack	Lunch	Snack	Dinner	Snack	Bedtime	Night	Notes
Blood Sugar									
Insulin Dose									
Grams Carb									
Activity									

Date:	Breakfast	Snack	Lunch	Snack	Dinner	Snack	Bedtime	Night	Notes
Blood Sugar									
Insulin Dose									
Grams Carb									
Activity									

Date:	Breakfast	Snack	Lunch	Snack	Dinner	Snack	Bedtime	Night	Notes
Blood Sugar									
Insulin Dose									
Grams Carb									
Activity									

Date:	Breakfast	Snack	Lunch	Snack	Dinner	Snack	Bedtime	Night	Notes
Blood Sugar									
Insulin Dose									
Grams Carb									
Activity									

Weekly Diabetes Record

Name: ______________________________

Date:	Breakfast	Snack	Lunch	Snack	Dinner	Snack	Bedtime	Night	Notes
Blood Sugar									
Insulin Dose									
Grams Carb									
Activity									

Date:	Breakfast	Snack	Lunch	Snack	Dinner	Snack	Bedtime	Night	Notes
Blood Sugar									
Insulin Dose									
Grams Carb									
Activity									

Date:	Breakfast	Snack	Lunch	Snack	Dinner	Snack	Bedtime	Night	Notes
Blood Sugar									
Insulin Dose									
Grams Carb									
Activity									

Date:	Breakfast	Snack	Lunch	Snack	Dinner	Snack	Bedtime	Night	Notes
Blood Sugar									
Insulin Dose									
Grams Carb									
Activity									

Date:	Breakfast	Snack	Lunch	Snack	Dinner	Snack	Bedtime	Night	Notes
Blood Sugar									
Insulin Dose									
Grams Carb									
Activity									

Date:	Breakfast	Snack	Lunch	Snack	Dinner	Snack	Bedtime	Night	Notes
Blood Sugar									
Insulin Dose									
Grams Carb									
Activity									

Date:	Breakfast	Snack	Lunch	Snack	Dinner	Snack	Bedtime	Night	Notes
Blood Sugar									
Insulin Dose									
Grams Carb									
Activity									

Weekly Diabetes Record

Name: ______________________________

Date:	Breakfast	Snack	Lunch	Snack	Dinner	Snack	Bedtime	Night	Notes
Blood Sugar									
Insulin Dose									
Grams Carb									
Activity									

Date:	Breakfast	Snack	Lunch	Snack	Dinner	Snack	Bedtime	Night	Notes
Blood Sugar									
Insulin Dose									
Grams Carb									
Activity									

Date:	Breakfast	Snack	Lunch	Snack	Dinner	Snack	Bedtime	Night	Notes
Blood Sugar									
Insulin Dose									
Grams Carb									
Activity									

Date:	Breakfast	Snack	Lunch	Snack	Dinner	Snack	Bedtime	Night	Notes
Blood Sugar									
Insulin Dose									
Grams Carb									
Activity									

Date:	Breakfast	Snack	Lunch	Snack	Dinner	Snack	Bedtime	Night	Notes
Blood Sugar									
Insulin Dose									
Grams Carb									
Activity									

Date:	Breakfast	Snack	Lunch	Snack	Dinner	Snack	Bedtime	Night	Notes
Blood Sugar									
Insulin Dose									
Grams Carb									
Activity									

Date:	Breakfast	Snack	Lunch	Snack	Dinner	Snack	Bedtime	Night	Notes
Blood Sugar									
Insulin Dose									
Grams Carb									
Activity									

Weekly Diabetes Record

Name: ____

Date:	Breakfast	Snack	Lunch	Snack	Dinner	Snack	Bedtime	Night	Notes
Blood Sugar									
Insulin Dose									
Grams Carb									
Activity									

Date:	Breakfast	Snack	Lunch	Snack	Dinner	Snack	Bedtime	Night	Notes
Blood Sugar									
Insulin Dose									
Grams Carb									
Activity									

Date:	Breakfast	Snack	Lunch	Snack	Dinner	Snack	Bedtime	Night	Notes
Blood Sugar									
Insulin Dose									
Grams Carb									
Activity									

Date:	Breakfast	Snack	Lunch	Snack	Dinner	Snack	Bedtime	Night	Notes
Blood Sugar									
Insulin Dose									
Grams Carb									
Activity									

Date:	Breakfast	Snack	Lunch	Snack	Dinner	Snack	Bedtime	Night	Notes
Blood Sugar									
Insulin Dose									
Grams Carb									
Activity									

Date:	Breakfast	Snack	Lunch	Snack	Dinner	Snack	Bedtime	Night	Notes
Blood Sugar									
Insulin Dose									
Grams Carb									
Activity									

Date:	Breakfast	Snack	Lunch	Snack	Dinner	Snack	Bedtime	Night	Notes
Blood Sugar									
Insulin Dose									
Grams Carb									
Activity									

Weekly Diabetes Record

Name: ______________________________

Date:	Breakfast	Snack	Lunch	Snack	Dinner	Snack	Bedtime	Night	Notes
Blood Sugar									
Insulin Dose									
Grams Carb									
Activity									

Date:	Breakfast	Snack	Lunch	Snack	Dinner	Snack	Bedtime	Night	Notes
Blood Sugar									
Insulin Dose									
Grams Carb									
Activity									

Date:	Breakfast	Snack	Lunch	Snack	Dinner	Snack	Bedtime	Night	Notes
Blood Sugar									
Insulin Dose									
Grams Carb									
Activity									

Date:	Breakfast	Snack	Lunch	Snack	Dinner	Snack	Bedtime	Night	Notes
Blood Sugar									
Insulin Dose									
Grams Carb									
Activity									

Date:	Breakfast	Snack	Lunch	Snack	Dinner	Snack	Bedtime	Night	Notes
Blood Sugar									
Insulin Dose									
Grams Carb									
Activity									

Date:	Breakfast	Snack	Lunch	Snack	Dinner	Snack	Bedtime	Night	Notes
Blood Sugar									
Insulin Dose									
Grams Carb									
Activity									

Date:	Breakfast	Snack	Lunch	Snack	Dinner	Snack	Bedtime	Night	Notes
Blood Sugar									
Insulin Dose									
Grams Carb									
Activity									

Weekly Diabetes Record

Name: ______________________________

Date:	Breakfast	Snack	Lunch	Snack	Dinner	Snack	Bedtime	Night	Notes
Blood Sugar									
Insulin Dose									
Grams Carb									
Activity									

Date:	Breakfast	Snack	Lunch	Snack	Dinner	Snack	Bedtime	Night	Notes
Blood Sugar									
Insulin Dose									
Grams Carb									
Activity									

Date:	Breakfast	Snack	Lunch	Snack	Dinner	Snack	Bedtime	Night	Notes
Blood Sugar									
Insulin Dose									
Grams Carb									
Activity									

Date:	Breakfast	Snack	Lunch	Snack	Dinner	Snack	Bedtime	Night	Notes
Blood Sugar									
Insulin Dose									
Grams Carb									
Activity									

Date:	Breakfast	Snack	Lunch	Snack	Dinner	Snack	Bedtime	Night	Notes
Blood Sugar									
Insulin Dose									
Grams Carb									
Activity									

Date:	Breakfast	Snack	Lunch	Snack	Dinner	Snack	Bedtime	Night	Notes
Blood Sugar									
Insulin Dose									
Grams Carb									
Activity									

Date:	Breakfast	Snack	Lunch	Snack	Dinner	Snack	Bedtime	Night	Notes
Blood Sugar									
Insulin Dose									
Grams Carb									
Activity									

Weekly Diabetes Record

Name: ____

Date:	Breakfast	Snack	Lunch	Snack	Dinner	Snack	Bedtime	Night	Notes
Blood Sugar									
Insulin Dose									
Grams Carb									
Activity									

Date:	Breakfast	Snack	Lunch	Snack	Dinner	Snack	Bedtime	Night	Notes
Blood Sugar									
Insulin Dose									
Grams Carb									
Activity									

Date:	Breakfast	Snack	Lunch	Snack	Dinner	Snack	Bedtime	Night	Notes
Blood Sugar									
Insulin Dose									
Grams Carb									
Activity									

Date:	Breakfast	Snack	Lunch	Snack	Dinner	Snack	Bedtime	Night	Notes
Blood Sugar									
Insulin Dose									
Grams Carb									
Activity									

Date:	Breakfast	Snack	Lunch	Snack	Dinner	Snack	Bedtime	Night	Notes
Blood Sugar									
Insulin Dose									
Grams Carb									
Activity									

Date:	Breakfast	Snack	Lunch	Snack	Dinner	Snack	Bedtime	Night	Notes
Blood Sugar									
Insulin Dose									
Grams Carb									
Activity									

Date:	Breakfast	Snack	Lunch	Snack	Dinner	Snack	Bedtime	Night	Notes
Blood Sugar									
Insulin Dose									
Grams Carb									
Activity									

Weekly Diabetes Record

Name: ____

Date:	Breakfast	Snack	Lunch	Snack	Dinner	Snack	Bedtime	Night	Notes
Blood Sugar									
Insulin Dose									
Grams Carb									
Activity									

Date:	Breakfast	Snack	Lunch	Snack	Dinner	Snack	Bedtime	Night	Notes
Blood Sugar									
Insulin Dose									
Grams Carb									
Activity									

Date:	Breakfast	Snack	Lunch	Snack	Dinner	Snack	Bedtime	Night	Notes
Blood Sugar									
Insulin Dose									
Grams Carb									
Activity									

Date:	Breakfast	Snack	Lunch	Snack	Dinner	Snack	Bedtime	Night	Notes
Blood Sugar									
Insulin Dose									
Grams Carb									
Activity									

Date:	Breakfast	Snack	Lunch	Snack	Dinner	Snack	Bedtime	Night	Notes
Blood Sugar									
Insulin Dose									
Grams Carb									
Activity									

Date:	Breakfast	Snack	Lunch	Snack	Dinner	Snack	Bedtime	Night	Notes
Blood Sugar									
Insulin Dose									
Grams Carb									
Activity									

Date:	Breakfast	Snack	Lunch	Snack	Dinner	Snack	Bedtime	Night	Notes
Blood Sugar									
Insulin Dose									
Grams Carb									
Activity									

Weekly Diabetes Record

Name: ______________________________

Date:	Breakfast	Snack	Lunch	Snack	Dinner	Snack	Bedtime	Night	Notes
Blood Sugar									
Insulin Dose									
Grams Carb									
Activity									

Date:	Breakfast	Snack	Lunch	Snack	Dinner	Snack	Bedtime	Night	Notes
Blood Sugar									
Insulin Dose									
Grams Carb									
Activity									

Date:	Breakfast	Snack	Lunch	Snack	Dinner	Snack	Bedtime	Night	Notes
Blood Sugar									
Insulin Dose									
Grams Carb									
Activity									

Date:	Breakfast	Snack	Lunch	Snack	Dinner	Snack	Bedtime	Night	Notes
Blood Sugar									
Insulin Dose									
Grams Carb									
Activity									

Date:	Breakfast	Snack	Lunch	Snack	Dinner	Snack	Bedtime	Night	Notes
Blood Sugar									
Insulin Dose									
Grams Carb									
Activity									

Date:	Breakfast	Snack	Lunch	Snack	Dinner	Snack	Bedtime	Night	Notes
Blood Sugar									
Insulin Dose									
Grams Carb									
Activity									

Date:	Breakfast	Snack	Lunch	Snack	Dinner	Snack	Bedtime	Night	Notes
Blood Sugar									
Insulin Dose									
Grams Carb									
Activity									

Weekly Diabetes Record

Name: ____________________________________

Date:	Breakfast	Snack	Lunch	Snack	Dinner	Snack	Bedtime	Night	Notes
Blood Sugar									
Insulin Dose									
Grams Carb									
Activity									

Date:	Breakfast	Snack	Lunch	Snack	Dinner	Snack	Bedtime	Night	Notes
Blood Sugar									
Insulin Dose									
Grams Carb									
Activity									

Date:	Breakfast	Snack	Lunch	Snack	Dinner	Snack	Bedtime	Night	Notes
Blood Sugar									
Insulin Dose									
Grams Carb									
Activity									

Date:	Breakfast	Snack	Lunch	Snack	Dinner	Snack	Bedtime	Night	Notes
Blood Sugar									
Insulin Dose									
Grams Carb									
Activity									

Date:	Breakfast	Snack	Lunch	Snack	Dinner	Snack	Bedtime	Night	Notes
Blood Sugar									
Insulin Dose									
Grams Carb									
Activity									

Date:	Breakfast	Snack	Lunch	Snack	Dinner	Snack	Bedtime	Night	Notes
Blood Sugar									
Insulin Dose									
Grams Carb									
Activity									

Date:	Breakfast	Snack	Lunch	Snack	Dinner	Snack	Bedtime	Night	Notes
Blood Sugar									
Insulin Dose									
Grams Carb									
Activity									

Weekly Diabetes Record

Name: ______________________________

Date:	Breakfast	Snack	Lunch	Snack	Dinner	Snack	Bedtime	Night	Notes
Blood Sugar									
Insulin Dose									
Grams Carb									
Activity									

Date:	Breakfast	Snack	Lunch	Snack	Dinner	Snack	Bedtime	Night	Notes
Blood Sugar									
Insulin Dose									
Grams Carb									
Activity									

Date:	Breakfast	Snack	Lunch	Snack	Dinner	Snack	Bedtime	Night	Notes
Blood Sugar									
Insulin Dose									
Grams Carb									
Activity									

Date:	Breakfast	Snack	Lunch	Snack	Dinner	Snack	Bedtime	Night	Notes
Blood Sugar									
Insulin Dose									
Grams Carb									
Activity									

Date:	Breakfast	Snack	Lunch	Snack	Dinner	Snack	Bedtime	Night	Notes
Blood Sugar									
Insulin Dose									
Grams Carb									
Activity									

Date:	Breakfast	Snack	Lunch	Snack	Dinner	Snack	Bedtime	Night	Notes
Blood Sugar									
Insulin Dose									
Grams Carb									
Activity									

Date:	Breakfast	Snack	Lunch	Snack	Dinner	Snack	Bedtime	Night	Notes
Blood Sugar									
Insulin Dose									
Grams Carb									
Activity									

Weekly Diabetes Record

Name: ______________________________

Date:	Breakfast	Snack	Lunch	Snack	Dinner	Snack	Bedtime	Night	Notes
Blood Sugar									
Insulin Dose									
Grams Carb									
Activity									

Date:	Breakfast	Snack	Lunch	Snack	Dinner	Snack	Bedtime	Night	Notes
Blood Sugar									
Insulin Dose									
Grams Carb									
Activity									

Date:	Breakfast	Snack	Lunch	Snack	Dinner	Snack	Bedtime	Night	Notes
Blood Sugar									
Insulin Dose									
Grams Carb									
Activity									

Date:	Breakfast	Snack	Lunch	Snack	Dinner	Snack	Bedtime	Night	Notes
Blood Sugar									
Insulin Dose									
Grams Carb									
Activity									

Date:	Breakfast	Snack	Lunch	Snack	Dinner	Snack	Bedtime	Night	Notes
Blood Sugar									
Insulin Dose									
Grams Carb									
Activity									

Date:	Breakfast	Snack	Lunch	Snack	Dinner	Snack	Bedtime	Night	Notes
Blood Sugar									
Insulin Dose									
Grams Carb									
Activity									

Date:	Breakfast	Snack	Lunch	Snack	Dinner	Snack	Bedtime	Night	Notes
Blood Sugar									
Insulin Dose									
Grams Carb									
Activity									

Weekly Diabetes Record

Name: ____

Date:	Breakfast	Snack	Lunch	Snack	Dinner	Snack	Bedtime	Night	Notes
Blood Sugar									
Insulin Dose									
Grams Carb									
Activity									

Date:	Breakfast	Snack	Lunch	Snack	Dinner	Snack	Bedtime	Night	Notes
Blood Sugar									
Insulin Dose									
Grams Carb									
Activity									

Date:	Breakfast	Snack	Lunch	Snack	Dinner	Snack	Bedtime	Night	Notes
Blood Sugar									
Insulin Dose									
Grams Carb									
Activity									

Date:	Breakfast	Snack	Lunch	Snack	Dinner	Snack	Bedtime	Night	Notes
Blood Sugar									
Insulin Dose									
Grams Carb									
Activity									

Date:	Breakfast	Snack	Lunch	Snack	Dinner	Snack	Bedtime	Night	Notes
Blood Sugar									
Insulin Dose									
Grams Carb									
Activity									

Date:	Breakfast	Snack	Lunch	Snack	Dinner	Snack	Bedtime	Night	Notes
Blood Sugar									
Insulin Dose									
Grams Carb									
Activity									

Date:	Breakfast	Snack	Lunch	Snack	Dinner	Snack	Bedtime	Night	Notes
Blood Sugar									
Insulin Dose									
Grams Carb									
Activity									

Weekly Diabetes Record

Name: ______________________________

Date:	Breakfast	Snack	Lunch	Snack	Dinner	Snack	Bedtime	Night	Notes
Blood Sugar									
Insulin Dose									
Grams Carb									
Activity									

Date:	Breakfast	Snack	Lunch	Snack	Dinner	Snack	Bedtime	Night	Notes
Blood Sugar									
Insulin Dose									
Grams Carb									
Activity									

Date:	Breakfast	Snack	Lunch	Snack	Dinner	Snack	Bedtime	Night	Notes
Blood Sugar									
Insulin Dose									
Grams Carb									
Activity									

Date:	Breakfast	Snack	Lunch	Snack	Dinner	Snack	Bedtime	Night	Notes
Blood Sugar									
Insulin Dose									
Grams Carb									
Activity									

Date:	Breakfast	Snack	Lunch	Snack	Dinner	Snack	Bedtime	Night	Notes
Blood Sugar									
Insulin Dose									
Grams Carb									
Activity									

Date:	Breakfast	Snack	Lunch	Snack	Dinner	Snack	Bedtime	Night	Notes
Blood Sugar									
Insulin Dose									
Grams Carb									
Activity									

Date:	Breakfast	Snack	Lunch	Snack	Dinner	Snack	Bedtime	Night	Notes
Blood Sugar									
Insulin Dose									
Grams Carb									
Activity									

Weekly Diabetes Record

Name: ____________________

Date:	Breakfast	Snack	Lunch	Snack	Dinner	Snack	Bedtime	Night	Notes
Blood Sugar									
Insulin Dose									
Grams Carb									
Activity									

Date:	Breakfast	Snack	Lunch	Snack	Dinner	Snack	Bedtime	Night	Notes
Blood Sugar									
Insulin Dose									
Grams Carb									
Activity									

Date:	Breakfast	Snack	Lunch	Snack	Dinner	Snack	Bedtime	Night	Notes
Blood Sugar									
Insulin Dose									
Grams Carb									
Activity									

Date:	Breakfast	Snack	Lunch	Snack	Dinner	Snack	Bedtime	Night	Notes
Blood Sugar									
Insulin Dose									
Grams Carb									
Activity									

Date:	Breakfast	Snack	Lunch	Snack	Dinner	Snack	Bedtime	Night	Notes
Blood Sugar									
Insulin Dose									
Grams Carb									
Activity									

Date:	Breakfast	Snack	Lunch	Snack	Dinner	Snack	Bedtime	Night	Notes
Blood Sugar									
Insulin Dose									
Grams Carb									
Activity									

Date:	Breakfast	Snack	Lunch	Snack	Dinner	Snack	Bedtime	Night	Notes
Blood Sugar									
Insulin Dose									
Grams Carb									
Activity									

Weekly Diabetes Record

Name: ______________________________

Date:	Breakfast	Snack	Lunch	Snack	Dinner	Snack	Bedtime	Night	Notes
Blood Sugar									
Insulin Dose									
Grams Carb									
Activity									

Date:	Breakfast	Snack	Lunch	Snack	Dinner	Snack	Bedtime	Night	Notes
Blood Sugar									
Insulin Dose									
Grams Carb									
Activity									

Date:	Breakfast	Snack	Lunch	Snack	Dinner	Snack	Bedtime	Night	Notes
Blood Sugar									
Insulin Dose									
Grams Carb									
Activity									

Date:	Breakfast	Snack	Lunch	Snack	Dinner	Snack	Bedtime	Night	Notes
Blood Sugar									
Insulin Dose									
Grams Carb									
Activity									

Date:	Breakfast	Snack	Lunch	Snack	Dinner	Snack	Bedtime	Night	Notes
Blood Sugar									
Insulin Dose									
Grams Carb									
Activity									

Date:	Breakfast	Snack	Lunch	Snack	Dinner	Snack	Bedtime	Night	Notes
Blood Sugar									
Insulin Dose									
Grams Carb									
Activity									

Date:	Breakfast	Snack	Lunch	Snack	Dinner	Snack	Bedtime	Night	Notes
Blood Sugar									
Insulin Dose									
Grams Carb									
Activity									

Weekly Diabetes Record

Name: ______________________________

Date:	Breakfast	Snack	Lunch	Snack	Dinner	Snack	Bedtime	Night	Notes
Blood Sugar									
Insulin Dose									
Grams Carb									
Activity									

Date:	Breakfast	Snack	Lunch	Snack	Dinner	Snack	Bedtime	Night	Notes
Blood Sugar									
Insulin Dose									
Grams Carb									
Activity									

Date:	Breakfast	Snack	Lunch	Snack	Dinner	Snack	Bedtime	Night	Notes
Blood Sugar									
Insulin Dose									
Grams Carb									
Activity									

Date:	Breakfast	Snack	Lunch	Snack	Dinner	Snack	Bedtime	Night	Notes
Blood Sugar									
Insulin Dose									
Grams Carb									
Activity									

Date:	Breakfast	Snack	Lunch	Snack	Dinner	Snack	Bedtime	Night	Notes
Blood Sugar									
Insulin Dose									
Grams Carb									
Activity									

Date:	Breakfast	Snack	Lunch	Snack	Dinner	Snack	Bedtime	Night	Notes
Blood Sugar									
Insulin Dose									
Grams Carb									
Activity									

Date:	Breakfast	Snack	Lunch	Snack	Dinner	Snack	Bedtime	Night	Notes
Blood Sugar									
Insulin Dose									
Grams Carb									
Activity									

Weekly Diabetes Record

Name: ______________________________

Date:	Breakfast	Snack	Lunch	Snack	Dinner	Snack	Bedtime	Night	Notes
Blood Sugar									
Insulin Dose									
Grams Carb									
Activity									

Date:	Breakfast	Snack	Lunch	Snack	Dinner	Snack	Bedtime	Night	Notes
Blood Sugar									
Insulin Dose									
Grams Carb									
Activity									

Date:	Breakfast	Snack	Lunch	Snack	Dinner	Snack	Bedtime	Night	Notes
Blood Sugar									
Insulin Dose									
Grams Carb									
Activity									

Date:	Breakfast	Snack	Lunch	Snack	Dinner	Snack	Bedtime	Night	Notes
Blood Sugar									
Insulin Dose									
Grams Carb									
Activity									

Date:	Breakfast	Snack	Lunch	Snack	Dinner	Snack	Bedtime	Night	Notes
Blood Sugar									
Insulin Dose									
Grams Carb									
Activity									

Date:	Breakfast	Snack	Lunch	Snack	Dinner	Snack	Bedtime	Night	Notes
Blood Sugar									
Insulin Dose									
Grams Carb									
Activity									

Date:	Breakfast	Snack	Lunch	Snack	Dinner	Snack	Bedtime	Night	Notes
Blood Sugar									
Insulin Dose									
Grams Carb									
Activity									

Weekly Diabetes Record

Name: ______________________________

Date:	Breakfast	Snack	Lunch	Snack	Dinner	Snack	Bedtime	Night	Notes
Blood Sugar									
Insulin Dose									
Grams Carb									
Activity									

Date:	Breakfast	Snack	Lunch	Snack	Dinner	Snack	Bedtime	Night	Notes
Blood Sugar									
Insulin Dose									
Grams Carb									
Activity									

Date:	Breakfast	Snack	Lunch	Snack	Dinner	Snack	Bedtime	Night	Notes
Blood Sugar									
Insulin Dose									
Grams Carb									
Activity									

Date:	Breakfast	Snack	Lunch	Snack	Dinner	Snack	Bedtime	Night	Notes
Blood Sugar									
Insulin Dose									
Grams Carb									
Activity									

Date:	Breakfast	Snack	Lunch	Snack	Dinner	Snack	Bedtime	Night	Notes
Blood Sugar									
Insulin Dose									
Grams Carb									
Activity									

Date:	Breakfast	Snack	Lunch	Snack	Dinner	Snack	Bedtime	Night	Notes
Blood Sugar									
Insulin Dose									
Grams Carb									
Activity									

Date:	Breakfast	Snack	Lunch	Snack	Dinner	Snack	Bedtime	Night	Notes
Blood Sugar									
Insulin Dose									
Grams Carb									
Activity									

Weekly Diabetes Record

Name: ______________________________

Date:	Breakfast	Snack	Lunch	Snack	Dinner	Snack	Bedtime	Night	Notes
Blood Sugar									
Insulin Dose									
Grams Carb									
Activity									

Date:	Breakfast	Snack	Lunch	Snack	Dinner	Snack	Bedtime	Night	Notes
Blood Sugar									
Insulin Dose									
Grams Carb									
Activity									

Date:	Breakfast	Snack	Lunch	Snack	Dinner	Snack	Bedtime	Night	Notes
Blood Sugar									
Insulin Dose									
Grams Carb									
Activity									

Date:	Breakfast	Snack	Lunch	Snack	Dinner	Snack	Bedtime	Night	Notes
Blood Sugar									
Insulin Dose									
Grams Carb									
Activity									

Date:	Breakfast	Snack	Lunch	Snack	Dinner	Snack	Bedtime	Night	Notes
Blood Sugar									
Insulin Dose									
Grams Carb									
Activity									

Date:	Breakfast	Snack	Lunch	Snack	Dinner	Snack	Bedtime	Night	Notes
Blood Sugar									
Insulin Dose									
Grams Carb									
Activity									

Date:	Breakfast	Snack	Lunch	Snack	Dinner	Snack	Bedtime	Night	Notes
Blood Sugar									
Insulin Dose									
Grams Carb									
Activity									

Weekly Diabetes Record

Name: ______________________________

Date:	Breakfast	Snack	Lunch	Snack	Dinner	Snack	Bedtime	Night	Notes
Blood Sugar									
Insulin Dose									
Grams Carb									
Activity									

Date:	Breakfast	Snack	Lunch	Snack	Dinner	Snack	Bedtime	Night	Notes
Blood Sugar									
Insulin Dose									
Grams Carb									
Activity									

Date:	Breakfast	Snack	Lunch	Snack	Dinner	Snack	Bedtime	Night	Notes
Blood Sugar									
Insulin Dose									
Grams Carb									
Activity									

Date:	Breakfast	Snack	Lunch	Snack	Dinner	Snack	Bedtime	Night	Notes
Blood Sugar									
Insulin Dose									
Grams Carb									
Activity									

Date:	Breakfast	Snack	Lunch	Snack	Dinner	Snack	Bedtime	Night	Notes
Blood Sugar									
Insulin Dose									
Grams Carb									
Activity									

Date:	Breakfast	Snack	Lunch	Snack	Dinner	Snack	Bedtime	Night	Notes
Blood Sugar									
Insulin Dose									
Grams Carb									
Activity									

Date:	Breakfast	Snack	Lunch	Snack	Dinner	Snack	Bedtime	Night	Notes
Blood Sugar									
Insulin Dose									
Grams Carb									
Activity									

Weekly Diabetes Record

Name: ______________________________

Date:	Breakfast	Snack	Lunch	Snack	Dinner	Snack	Bedtime	Night	Notes
Blood Sugar									
Insulin Dose									
Grams Carb									
Activity									

Date:	Breakfast	Snack	Lunch	Snack	Dinner	Snack	Bedtime	Night	Notes
Blood Sugar									
Insulin Dose									
Grams Carb									
Activity									

Date:	Breakfast	Snack	Lunch	Snack	Dinner	Snack	Bedtime	Night	Notes
Blood Sugar									
Insulin Dose									
Grams Carb									
Activity									

Date:	Breakfast	Snack	Lunch	Snack	Dinner	Snack	Bedtime	Night	Notes
Blood Sugar									
Insulin Dose									
Grams Carb									
Activity									

Date:	Breakfast	Snack	Lunch	Snack	Dinner	Snack	Bedtime	Night	Notes
Blood Sugar									
Insulin Dose									
Grams Carb									
Activity									

Date:	Breakfast	Snack	Lunch	Snack	Dinner	Snack	Bedtime	Night	Notes
Blood Sugar									
Insulin Dose									
Grams Carb									
Activity									

Date:	Breakfast	Snack	Lunch	Snack	Dinner	Snack	Bedtime	Night	Notes
Blood Sugar									
Insulin Dose									
Grams Carb									
Activity									

Weekly Diabetes Record

Name: ______________________________

Date:	Breakfast	Snack	Lunch	Snack	Dinner	Snack	Bedtime	Night	Notes
Blood Sugar									
Insulin Dose									
Grams Carb									
Activity									

Date:	Breakfast	Snack	Lunch	Snack	Dinner	Snack	Bedtime	Night	Notes
Blood Sugar									
Insulin Dose									
Grams Carb									
Activity									

Date:	Breakfast	Snack	Lunch	Snack	Dinner	Snack	Bedtime	Night	Notes
Blood Sugar									
Insulin Dose									
Grams Carb									
Activity									

Date:	Breakfast	Snack	Lunch	Snack	Dinner	Snack	Bedtime	Night	Notes
Blood Sugar									
Insulin Dose									
Grams Carb									
Activity									

Date:	Breakfast	Snack	Lunch	Snack	Dinner	Snack	Bedtime	Night	Notes
Blood Sugar									
Insulin Dose									
Grams Carb									
Activity									

Date:	Breakfast	Snack	Lunch	Snack	Dinner	Snack	Bedtime	Night	Notes
Blood Sugar									
Insulin Dose									
Grams Carb									
Activity									

Date:	Breakfast	Snack	Lunch	Snack	Dinner	Snack	Bedtime	Night	Notes
Blood Sugar									
Insulin Dose									
Grams Carb									
Activity									

Weekly Diabetes Record

Name: ____

Date:	Breakfast	Snack	Lunch	Snack	Dinner	Snack	Bedtime	Night	Notes
Blood Sugar									
Insulin Dose									
Grams Carb									
Activity									

Date:	Breakfast	Snack	Lunch	Snack	Dinner	Snack	Bedtime	Night	Notes
Blood Sugar									
Insulin Dose									
Grams Carb									
Activity									

Date:	Breakfast	Snack	Lunch	Snack	Dinner	Snack	Bedtime	Night	Notes
Blood Sugar									
Insulin Dose									
Grams Carb									
Activity									

Date:	Breakfast	Snack	Lunch	Snack	Dinner	Snack	Bedtime	Night	Notes
Blood Sugar									
Insulin Dose									
Grams Carb									
Activity									

Date:	Breakfast	Snack	Lunch	Snack	Dinner	Snack	Bedtime	Night	Notes
Blood Sugar									
Insulin Dose									
Grams Carb									
Activity									

Date:	Breakfast	Snack	Lunch	Snack	Dinner	Snack	Bedtime	Night	Notes
Blood Sugar									
Insulin Dose									
Grams Carb									
Activity									

Date:	Breakfast	Snack	Lunch	Snack	Dinner	Snack	Bedtime	Night	Notes
Blood Sugar									
Insulin Dose									
Grams Carb									
Activity									

Weekly Diabetes Record

Name: ______________________________

Date:	Breakfast	Snack	Lunch	Snack	Dinner	Snack	Bedtime	Night	Notes
Blood Sugar									
Insulin Dose									
Grams Carb									
Activity									

Date:	Breakfast	Snack	Lunch	Snack	Dinner	Snack	Bedtime	Night	Notes
Blood Sugar									
Insulin Dose									
Grams Carb									
Activity									

Date:	Breakfast	Snack	Lunch	Snack	Dinner	Snack	Bedtime	Night	Notes
Blood Sugar									
Insulin Dose									
Grams Carb									
Activity									

Date:	Breakfast	Snack	Lunch	Snack	Dinner	Snack	Bedtime	Night	Notes
Blood Sugar									
Insulin Dose									
Grams Carb									
Activity									

Date:	Breakfast	Snack	Lunch	Snack	Dinner	Snack	Bedtime	Night	Notes
Blood Sugar									
Insulin Dose									
Grams Carb									
Activity									

Date:	Breakfast	Snack	Lunch	Snack	Dinner	Snack	Bedtime	Night	Notes
Blood Sugar									
Insulin Dose									
Grams Carb									
Activity									

Date:	Breakfast	Snack	Lunch	Snack	Dinner	Snack	Bedtime	Night	Notes
Blood Sugar									
Insulin Dose									
Grams Carb									
Activity									

Weekly Diabetes Record

Name: ______________________________

Date:	Breakfast	Snack	Lunch	Snack	Dinner	Snack	Bedtime	Night	Notes
Blood Sugar									
Insulin Dose									
Grams Carb									
Activity									

Date:	Breakfast	Snack	Lunch	Snack	Dinner	Snack	Bedtime	Night	Notes
Blood Sugar									
Insulin Dose									
Grams Carb									
Activity									

Date:	Breakfast	Snack	Lunch	Snack	Dinner	Snack	Bedtime	Night	Notes
Blood Sugar									
Insulin Dose									
Grams Carb									
Activity									

Date:	Breakfast	Snack	Lunch	Snack	Dinner	Snack	Bedtime	Night	Notes
Blood Sugar									
Insulin Dose									
Grams Carb									
Activity									

Date:	Breakfast	Snack	Lunch	Snack	Dinner	Snack	Bedtime	Night	Notes
Blood Sugar									
Insulin Dose									
Grams Carb									
Activity									

Date:	Breakfast	Snack	Lunch	Snack	Dinner	Snack	Bedtime	Night	Notes
Blood Sugar									
Insulin Dose									
Grams Carb									
Activity									

Date:	Breakfast	Snack	Lunch	Snack	Dinner	Snack	Bedtime	Night	Notes
Blood Sugar									
Insulin Dose									
Grams Carb									
Activity									

Weekly Diabetes Record

Name: ______________________________

Date:	Breakfast	Snack	Lunch	Snack	Dinner	Snack	Bedtime	Night	Notes
Blood Sugar									
Insulin Dose									
Grams Carb									
Activity									

Date:	Breakfast	Snack	Lunch	Snack	Dinner	Snack	Bedtime	Night	Notes
Blood Sugar									
Insulin Dose									
Grams Carb									
Activity									

Date:	Breakfast	Snack	Lunch	Snack	Dinner	Snack	Bedtime	Night	Notes
Blood Sugar									
Insulin Dose									
Grams Carb									
Activity									

Date:	Breakfast	Snack	Lunch	Snack	Dinner	Snack	Bedtime	Night	Notes
Blood Sugar									
Insulin Dose									
Grams Carb									
Activity									

Date:	Breakfast	Snack	Lunch	Snack	Dinner	Snack	Bedtime	Night	Notes
Blood Sugar									
Insulin Dose									
Grams Carb									
Activity									

Date:	Breakfast	Snack	Lunch	Snack	Dinner	Snack	Bedtime	Night	Notes
Blood Sugar									
Insulin Dose									
Grams Carb									
Activity									

Date:	Breakfast	Snack	Lunch	Snack	Dinner	Snack	Bedtime	Night	Notes
Blood Sugar									
Insulin Dose									
Grams Carb									
Activity									

Weekly Diabetes Record

Name: ____

Date:	Breakfast	Snack	Lunch	Snack	Dinner	Snack	Bedtime	Night	Notes
Blood Sugar									
Insulin Dose									
Grams Carb									
Activity									

Date:	Breakfast	Snack	Lunch	Snack	Dinner	Snack	Bedtime	Night	Notes
Blood Sugar									
Insulin Dose									
Grams Carb									
Activity									

Date:	Breakfast	Snack	Lunch	Snack	Dinner	Snack	Bedtime	Night	Notes
Blood Sugar									
Insulin Dose									
Grams Carb									
Activity									

Date:	Breakfast	Snack	Lunch	Snack	Dinner	Snack	Bedtime	Night	Notes
Blood Sugar									
Insulin Dose									
Grams Carb									
Activity									

Date:	Breakfast	Snack	Lunch	Snack	Dinner	Snack	Bedtime	Night	Notes
Blood Sugar									
Insulin Dose									
Grams Carb									
Activity									

Date:	Breakfast	Snack	Lunch	Snack	Dinner	Snack	Bedtime	Night	Notes
Blood Sugar									
Insulin Dose									
Grams Carb									
Activity									

Date:	Breakfast	Snack	Lunch	Snack	Dinner	Snack	Bedtime	Night	Notes
Blood Sugar									
Insulin Dose									
Grams Carb									
Activity									

Weekly Diabetes Record

Name: ______________________________

Date:	Breakfast	Snack	Lunch	Snack	Dinner	Snack	Bedtime	Night	Notes
Blood Sugar									
Insulin Dose									
Grams Carb									
Activity									

Date:	Breakfast	Snack	Lunch	Snack	Dinner	Snack	Bedtime	Night	Notes
Blood Sugar									
Insulin Dose									
Grams Carb									
Activity									

Date:	Breakfast	Snack	Lunch	Snack	Dinner	Snack	Bedtime	Night	Notes
Blood Sugar									
Insulin Dose									
Grams Carb									
Activity									

Date:	Breakfast	Snack	Lunch	Snack	Dinner	Snack	Bedtime	Night	Notes
Blood Sugar									
Insulin Dose									
Grams Carb									
Activity									

Date:	Breakfast	Snack	Lunch	Snack	Dinner	Snack	Bedtime	Night	Notes
Blood Sugar									
Insulin Dose									
Grams Carb									
Activity									

Date:	Breakfast	Snack	Lunch	Snack	Dinner	Snack	Bedtime	Night	Notes
Blood Sugar									
Insulin Dose									
Grams Carb									
Activity									

Date:	Breakfast	Snack	Lunch	Snack	Dinner	Snack	Bedtime	Night	Notes
Blood Sugar									
Insulin Dose									
Grams Carb									
Activity									

Weekly Diabetes Record

Name: ______________________________

Date:	Breakfast	Snack	Lunch	Snack	Dinner	Snack	Bedtime	Night	Notes
Blood Sugar									
Insulin Dose									
Grams Carb									
Activity									

Date:	Breakfast	Snack	Lunch	Snack	Dinner	Snack	Bedtime	Night	Notes
Blood Sugar									
Insulin Dose									
Grams Carb									
Activity									

Date:	Breakfast	Snack	Lunch	Snack	Dinner	Snack	Bedtime	Night	Notes
Blood Sugar									
Insulin Dose									
Grams Carb									
Activity									

Date:	Breakfast	Snack	Lunch	Snack	Dinner	Snack	Bedtime	Night	Notes
Blood Sugar									
Insulin Dose									
Grams Carb									
Activity									

Date:	Breakfast	Snack	Lunch	Snack	Dinner	Snack	Bedtime	Night	Notes
Blood Sugar									
Insulin Dose									
Grams Carb									
Activity									

Date:	Breakfast	Snack	Lunch	Snack	Dinner	Snack	Bedtime	Night	Notes
Blood Sugar									
Insulin Dose									
Grams Carb									
Activity									

Date:	Breakfast	Snack	Lunch	Snack	Dinner	Snack	Bedtime	Night	Notes
Blood Sugar									
Insulin Dose									
Grams Carb									
Activity									

Weekly Diabetes Record

Name: ______________________________

Date:	Breakfast	Snack	Lunch	Snack	Dinner	Snack	Bedtime	Night	Notes
Blood Sugar									
Insulin Dose									
Grams Carb									
Activity									

Date:	Breakfast	Snack	Lunch	Snack	Dinner	Snack	Bedtime	Night	Notes
Blood Sugar									
Insulin Dose									
Grams Carb									
Activity									

Date:	Breakfast	Snack	Lunch	Snack	Dinner	Snack	Bedtime	Night	Notes
Blood Sugar									
Insulin Dose									
Grams Carb									
Activity									

Date:	Breakfast	Snack	Lunch	Snack	Dinner	Snack	Bedtime	Night	Notes
Blood Sugar									
Insulin Dose									
Grams Carb									
Activity									

Date:	Breakfast	Snack	Lunch	Snack	Dinner	Snack	Bedtime	Night	Notes
Blood Sugar									
Insulin Dose									
Grams Carb									
Activity									

Date:	Breakfast	Snack	Lunch	Snack	Dinner	Snack	Bedtime	Night	Notes
Blood Sugar									
Insulin Dose									
Grams Carb									
Activity									

Date:	Breakfast	Snack	Lunch	Snack	Dinner	Snack	Bedtime	Night	Notes
Blood Sugar									
Insulin Dose									
Grams Carb									
Activity									

Weekly Diabetes Record

Name: ______________________________

Date:	Breakfast	Snack	Lunch	Snack	Dinner	Snack	Bedtime	Night	Notes
Blood Sugar									
Insulin Dose									
Grams Carb									
Activity									

Date:	Breakfast	Snack	Lunch	Snack	Dinner	Snack	Bedtime	Night	Notes
Blood Sugar									
Insulin Dose									
Grams Carb									
Activity									

Date:	Breakfast	Snack	Lunch	Snack	Dinner	Snack	Bedtime	Night	Notes
Blood Sugar									
Insulin Dose									
Grams Carb									
Activity									

Date:	Breakfast	Snack	Lunch	Snack	Dinner	Snack	Bedtime	Night	Notes
Blood Sugar									
Insulin Dose									
Grams Carb									
Activity									

Date:	Breakfast	Snack	Lunch	Snack	Dinner	Snack	Bedtime	Night	Notes
Blood Sugar									
Insulin Dose									
Grams Carb									
Activity									

Date:	Breakfast	Snack	Lunch	Snack	Dinner	Snack	Bedtime	Night	Notes
Blood Sugar									
Insulin Dose									
Grams Carb									
Activity									

Date:	Breakfast	Snack	Lunch	Snack	Dinner	Snack	Bedtime	Night	Notes
Blood Sugar									
Insulin Dose									
Grams Carb									
Activity									

Weekly Diabetes Record

Name: ______________________________

Date:	Breakfast	Snack	Lunch	Snack	Dinner	Snack	Bedtime	Night	Notes
Blood Sugar									
Insulin Dose									
Grams Carb									
Activity									

Date:	Breakfast	Snack	Lunch	Snack	Dinner	Snack	Bedtime	Night	Notes
Blood Sugar									
Insulin Dose									
Grams Carb									
Activity									

Date:	Breakfast	Snack	Lunch	Snack	Dinner	Snack	Bedtime	Night	Notes
Blood Sugar									
Insulin Dose									
Grams Carb									
Activity									

Date:	Breakfast	Snack	Lunch	Snack	Dinner	Snack	Bedtime	Night	Notes
Blood Sugar									
Insulin Dose									
Grams Carb									
Activity									

Date:	Breakfast	Snack	Lunch	Snack	Dinner	Snack	Bedtime	Night	Notes
Blood Sugar									
Insulin Dose									
Grams Carb									
Activity									

Date:	Breakfast	Snack	Lunch	Snack	Dinner	Snack	Bedtime	Night	Notes
Blood Sugar									
Insulin Dose									
Grams Carb									
Activity									

Date:	Breakfast	Snack	Lunch	Snack	Dinner	Snack	Bedtime	Night	Notes
Blood Sugar									
Insulin Dose									
Grams Carb									
Activity									

Weekly Diabetes Record

Name: ______________________________

Date:	Breakfast	Snack	Lunch	Snack	Dinner	Snack	Bedtime	Night	Notes
Blood Sugar									
Insulin Dose									
Grams Carb									
Activity									

Date:	Breakfast	Snack	Lunch	Snack	Dinner	Snack	Bedtime	Night	Notes
Blood Sugar									
Insulin Dose									
Grams Carb									
Activity									

Date:	Breakfast	Snack	Lunch	Snack	Dinner	Snack	Bedtime	Night	Notes
Blood Sugar									
Insulin Dose									
Grams Carb									
Activity									

Date:	Breakfast	Snack	Lunch	Snack	Dinner	Snack	Bedtime	Night	Notes
Blood Sugar									
Insulin Dose									
Grams Carb									
Activity									

Date:	Breakfast	Snack	Lunch	Snack	Dinner	Snack	Bedtime	Night	Notes
Blood Sugar									
Insulin Dose									
Grams Carb									
Activity									

Date:	Breakfast	Snack	Lunch	Snack	Dinner	Snack	Bedtime	Night	Notes
Blood Sugar									
Insulin Dose									
Grams Carb									
Activity									

Date:	Breakfast	Snack	Lunch	Snack	Dinner	Snack	Bedtime	Night	Notes
Blood Sugar									
Insulin Dose									
Grams Carb									
Activity									

Weekly Diabetes Record

Name: ______________________________

Date:	Breakfast	Snack	Lunch	Snack	Dinner	Snack	Bedtime	Night	Notes
Blood Sugar									
Insulin Dose									
Grams Carb									
Activity									

Date:	Breakfast	Snack	Lunch	Snack	Dinner	Snack	Bedtime	Night	Notes
Blood Sugar									
Insulin Dose									
Grams Carb									
Activity									

Date:	Breakfast	Snack	Lunch	Snack	Dinner	Snack	Bedtime	Night	Notes
Blood Sugar									
Insulin Dose									
Grams Carb									
Activity									

Date:	Breakfast	Snack	Lunch	Snack	Dinner	Snack	Bedtime	Night	Notes
Blood Sugar									
Insulin Dose									
Grams Carb									
Activity									

Date:	Breakfast	Snack	Lunch	Snack	Dinner	Snack	Bedtime	Night	Notes
Blood Sugar									
Insulin Dose									
Grams Carb									
Activity									

Date:	Breakfast	Snack	Lunch	Snack	Dinner	Snack	Bedtime	Night	Notes
Blood Sugar									
Insulin Dose									
Grams Carb									
Activity									

Date:	Breakfast	Snack	Lunch	Snack	Dinner	Snack	Bedtime	Night	Notes
Blood Sugar									
Insulin Dose									
Grams Carb									
Activity									

Weekly Diabetes Record

Name: ______________________________

Date:	Breakfast	Snack	Lunch	Snack	Dinner	Snack	Bedtime	Night	Notes
Blood Sugar									
Insulin Dose									
Grams Carb									
Activity									

Date:	Breakfast	Snack	Lunch	Snack	Dinner	Snack	Bedtime	Night	Notes
Blood Sugar									
Insulin Dose									
Grams Carb									
Activity									

Date:	Breakfast	Snack	Lunch	Snack	Dinner	Snack	Bedtime	Night	Notes
Blood Sugar									
Insulin Dose									
Grams Carb									
Activity									

Date:	Breakfast	Snack	Lunch	Snack	Dinner	Snack	Bedtime	Night	Notes
Blood Sugar									
Insulin Dose									
Grams Carb									
Activity									

Date:	Breakfast	Snack	Lunch	Snack	Dinner	Snack	Bedtime	Night	Notes
Blood Sugar									
Insulin Dose									
Grams Carb									
Activity									

Date:	Breakfast	Snack	Lunch	Snack	Dinner	Snack	Bedtime	Night	Notes
Blood Sugar									
Insulin Dose									
Grams Carb									
Activity									

Date:	Breakfast	Snack	Lunch	Snack	Dinner	Snack	Bedtime	Night	Notes
Blood Sugar									
Insulin Dose									
Grams Carb									
Activity									

Weekly Diabetes Record

Name: ______________________________

Date:	Breakfast	Snack	Lunch	Snack	Dinner	Snack	Bedtime	Night	Notes
Blood Sugar									
Insulin Dose									
Grams Carb									
Activity									

Date:	Breakfast	Snack	Lunch	Snack	Dinner	Snack	Bedtime	Night	Notes
Blood Sugar									
Insulin Dose									
Grams Carb									
Activity									

Date:	Breakfast	Snack	Lunch	Snack	Dinner	Snack	Bedtime	Night	Notes
Blood Sugar									
Insulin Dose									
Grams Carb									
Activity									

Date:	Breakfast	Snack	Lunch	Snack	Dinner	Snack	Bedtime	Night	Notes
Blood Sugar									
Insulin Dose									
Grams Carb									
Activity									

Date:	Breakfast	Snack	Lunch	Snack	Dinner	Snack	Bedtime	Night	Notes
Blood Sugar									
Insulin Dose									
Grams Carb									
Activity									

Date:	Breakfast	Snack	Lunch	Snack	Dinner	Snack	Bedtime	Night	Notes
Blood Sugar									
Insulin Dose									
Grams Carb									
Activity									

Date:	Breakfast	Snack	Lunch	Snack	Dinner	Snack	Bedtime	Night	Notes
Blood Sugar									
Insulin Dose									
Grams Carb									
Activity									

Weekly Diabetes Record

Name: ______________________________

Date:	Breakfast	Snack	Lunch	Snack	Dinner	Snack	Bedtime	Night	Notes
Blood Sugar									
Insulin Dose									
Grams Carb									
Activity									

Date:	Breakfast	Snack	Lunch	Snack	Dinner	Snack	Bedtime	Night	Notes
Blood Sugar									
Insulin Dose									
Grams Carb									
Activity									

Date:	Breakfast	Snack	Lunch	Snack	Dinner	Snack	Bedtime	Night	Notes
Blood Sugar									
Insulin Dose									
Grams Carb									
Activity									

Date:	Breakfast	Snack	Lunch	Snack	Dinner	Snack	Bedtime	Night	Notes
Blood Sugar									
Insulin Dose									
Grams Carb									
Activity									

Date:	Breakfast	Snack	Lunch	Snack	Dinner	Snack	Bedtime	Night	Notes
Blood Sugar									
Insulin Dose									
Grams Carb									
Activity									

Date:	Breakfast	Snack	Lunch	Snack	Dinner	Snack	Bedtime	Night	Notes
Blood Sugar									
Insulin Dose									
Grams Carb									
Activity									

Date:	Breakfast	Snack	Lunch	Snack	Dinner	Snack	Bedtime	Night	Notes
Blood Sugar									
Insulin Dose									
Grams Carb									
Activity									

Weekly Diabetes Record

Name: ______________________________

Date:	Breakfast	Snack	Lunch	Snack	Dinner	Snack	Bedtime	Night	Notes
Blood Sugar									
Insulin Dose									
Grams Carb									
Activity									

Date:	Breakfast	Snack	Lunch	Snack	Dinner	Snack	Bedtime	Night	Notes
Blood Sugar									
Insulin Dose									
Grams Carb									
Activity									

Date:	Breakfast	Snack	Lunch	Snack	Dinner	Snack	Bedtime	Night	Notes
Blood Sugar									
Insulin Dose									
Grams Carb									
Activity									

Date:	Breakfast	Snack	Lunch	Snack	Dinner	Snack	Bedtime	Night	Notes
Blood Sugar									
Insulin Dose									
Grams Carb									
Activity									

Date:	Breakfast	Snack	Lunch	Snack	Dinner	Snack	Bedtime	Night	Notes
Blood Sugar									
Insulin Dose									
Grams Carb									
Activity									

Date:	Breakfast	Snack	Lunch	Snack	Dinner	Snack	Bedtime	Night	Notes
Blood Sugar									
Insulin Dose									
Grams Carb									
Activity									

Date:	Breakfast	Snack	Lunch	Snack	Dinner	Snack	Bedtime	Night	Notes
Blood Sugar									
Insulin Dose									
Grams Carb									
Activity									

Weekly Diabetes Record

Name: ______________________________

Date:	Breakfast	Snack	Lunch	Snack	Dinner	Snack	Bedtime	Night	Notes
Blood Sugar									
Insulin Dose									
Grams Carb									
Activity									

Date:	Breakfast	Snack	Lunch	Snack	Dinner	Snack	Bedtime	Night	Notes
Blood Sugar									
Insulin Dose									
Grams Carb									
Activity									

Date:	Breakfast	Snack	Lunch	Snack	Dinner	Snack	Bedtime	Night	Notes
Blood Sugar									
Insulin Dose									
Grams Carb									
Activity									

Date:	Breakfast	Snack	Lunch	Snack	Dinner	Snack	Bedtime	Night	Notes
Blood Sugar									
Insulin Dose									
Grams Carb									
Activity									

Date:	Breakfast	Snack	Lunch	Snack	Dinner	Snack	Bedtime	Night	Notes
Blood Sugar									
Insulin Dose									
Grams Carb									
Activity									

Date:	Breakfast	Snack	Lunch	Snack	Dinner	Snack	Bedtime	Night	Notes
Blood Sugar									
Insulin Dose									
Grams Carb									
Activity									

Date:	Breakfast	Snack	Lunch	Snack	Dinner	Snack	Bedtime	Night	Notes
Blood Sugar									
Insulin Dose									
Grams Carb									
Activity									

Weekly Diabetes Record

Name: ____

Date:	Breakfast	Snack	Lunch	Snack	Dinner	Snack	Bedtime	Night	Notes
Blood Sugar									
Insulin Dose									
Grams Carb									
Activity									

Date:	Breakfast	Snack	Lunch	Snack	Dinner	Snack	Bedtime	Night	Notes
Blood Sugar									
Insulin Dose									
Grams Carb									
Activity									

Date:	Breakfast	Snack	Lunch	Snack	Dinner	Snack	Bedtime	Night	Notes
Blood Sugar									
Insulin Dose									
Grams Carb									
Activity									

Date:	Breakfast	Snack	Lunch	Snack	Dinner	Snack	Bedtime	Night	Notes
Blood Sugar									
Insulin Dose									
Grams Carb									
Activity									

Date:	Breakfast	Snack	Lunch	Snack	Dinner	Snack	Bedtime	Night	Notes
Blood Sugar									
Insulin Dose									
Grams Carb									
Activity									

Date:	Breakfast	Snack	Lunch	Snack	Dinner	Snack	Bedtime	Night	Notes
Blood Sugar									
Insulin Dose									
Grams Carb									
Activity									

Date:	Breakfast	Snack	Lunch	Snack	Dinner	Snack	Bedtime	Night	Notes
Blood Sugar									
Insulin Dose									
Grams Carb									
Activity									

Weekly Diabetes Record

Name: ____________________

Date:	Breakfast	Snack	Lunch	Snack	Dinner	Snack	Bedtime	Night	Notes
Blood Sugar									
Insulin Dose									
Grams Carb									
Activity									

Date:	Breakfast	Snack	Lunch	Snack	Dinner	Snack	Bedtime	Night	Notes
Blood Sugar									
Insulin Dose									
Grams Carb									
Activity									

Date:	Breakfast	Snack	Lunch	Snack	Dinner	Snack	Bedtime	Night	Notes
Blood Sugar									
Insulin Dose									
Grams Carb									
Activity									

Date:	Breakfast	Snack	Lunch	Snack	Dinner	Snack	Bedtime	Night	Notes
Blood Sugar									
Insulin Dose									
Grams Carb									
Activity									

Date:	Breakfast	Snack	Lunch	Snack	Dinner	Snack	Bedtime	Night	Notes
Blood Sugar									
Insulin Dose									
Grams Carb									
Activity									

Date:	Breakfast	Snack	Lunch	Snack	Dinner	Snack	Bedtime	Night	Notes
Blood Sugar									
Insulin Dose									
Grams Carb									
Activity									

Date:	Breakfast	Snack	Lunch	Snack	Dinner	Snack	Bedtime	Night	Notes
Blood Sugar									
Insulin Dose									
Grams Carb									
Activity									

Weekly Diabetes Record

Name: ______________________________

Date:	Breakfast	Snack	Lunch	Snack	Dinner	Snack	Bedtime	Night	Notes
Blood Sugar									
Insulin Dose									
Grams Carb									
Activity									

Date:	Breakfast	Snack	Lunch	Snack	Dinner	Snack	Bedtime	Night	Notes
Blood Sugar									
Insulin Dose									
Grams Carb									
Activity									

Date:	Breakfast	Snack	Lunch	Snack	Dinner	Snack	Bedtime	Night	Notes
Blood Sugar									
Insulin Dose									
Grams Carb									
Activity									

Date:	Breakfast	Snack	Lunch	Snack	Dinner	Snack	Bedtime	Night	Notes
Blood Sugar									
Insulin Dose									
Grams Carb									
Activity									

Date:	Breakfast	Snack	Lunch	Snack	Dinner	Snack	Bedtime	Night	Notes
Blood Sugar									
Insulin Dose									
Grams Carb									
Activity									

Date:	Breakfast	Snack	Lunch	Snack	Dinner	Snack	Bedtime	Night	Notes
Blood Sugar									
Insulin Dose									
Grams Carb									
Activity									

Date:	Breakfast	Snack	Lunch	Snack	Dinner	Snack	Bedtime	Night	Notes
Blood Sugar									
Insulin Dose									
Grams Carb									
Activity									

Weekly Diabetes Record

Name: ______________________________

Date:	Breakfast	Snack	Lunch	Snack	Dinner	Snack	Bedtime	Night	Notes
Blood Sugar									
Insulin Dose									
Grams Carb									
Activity									

Date:	Breakfast	Snack	Lunch	Snack	Dinner	Snack	Bedtime	Night	Notes
Blood Sugar									
Insulin Dose									
Grams Carb									
Activity									

Date:	Breakfast	Snack	Lunch	Snack	Dinner	Snack	Bedtime	Night	Notes
Blood Sugar									
Insulin Dose									
Grams Carb									
Activity									

Date:	Breakfast	Snack	Lunch	Snack	Dinner	Snack	Bedtime	Night	Notes
Blood Sugar									
Insulin Dose									
Grams Carb									
Activity									

Date:	Breakfast	Snack	Lunch	Snack	Dinner	Snack	Bedtime	Night	Notes
Blood Sugar									
Insulin Dose									
Grams Carb									
Activity									

Date:	Breakfast	Snack	Lunch	Snack	Dinner	Snack	Bedtime	Night	Notes
Blood Sugar									
Insulin Dose									
Grams Carb									
Activity									

Date:	Breakfast	Snack	Lunch	Snack	Dinner	Snack	Bedtime	Night	Notes
Blood Sugar									
Insulin Dose									
Grams Carb									
Activity									

Weekly Diabetes Record

Name: ______________________________

Date:	Breakfast	Snack	Lunch	Snack	Dinner	Snack	Bedtime	Night	Notes
Blood Sugar									
Insulin Dose									
Grams Carb									
Activity									

Date:	Breakfast	Snack	Lunch	Snack	Dinner	Snack	Bedtime	Night	Notes
Blood Sugar									
Insulin Dose									
Grams Carb									
Activity									

Date:	Breakfast	Snack	Lunch	Snack	Dinner	Snack	Bedtime	Night	Notes
Blood Sugar									
Insulin Dose									
Grams Carb									
Activity									

Date:	Breakfast	Snack	Lunch	Snack	Dinner	Snack	Bedtime	Night	Notes
Blood Sugar									
Insulin Dose									
Grams Carb									
Activity									

Date:	Breakfast	Snack	Lunch	Snack	Dinner	Snack	Bedtime	Night	Notes
Blood Sugar									
Insulin Dose									
Grams Carb									
Activity									

Date:	Breakfast	Snack	Lunch	Snack	Dinner	Snack	Bedtime	Night	Notes
Blood Sugar									
Insulin Dose									
Grams Carb									
Activity									

Date:	Breakfast	Snack	Lunch	Snack	Dinner	Snack	Bedtime	Night	Notes
Blood Sugar									
Insulin Dose									
Grams Carb									
Activity									

Weekly Diabetes Record

Name: ____

Date:	Breakfast	Snack	Lunch	Snack	Dinner	Snack	Bedtime	Night	Notes
Blood Sugar									
Insulin Dose									
Grams Carb									
Activity									

Date:	Breakfast	Snack	Lunch	Snack	Dinner	Snack	Bedtime	Night	Notes
Blood Sugar									
Insulin Dose									
Grams Carb									
Activity									

Date:	Breakfast	Snack	Lunch	Snack	Dinner	Snack	Bedtime	Night	Notes
Blood Sugar									
Insulin Dose									
Grams Carb									
Activity									

Date:	Breakfast	Snack	Lunch	Snack	Dinner	Snack	Bedtime	Night	Notes
Blood Sugar									
Insulin Dose									
Grams Carb									
Activity									

Date:	Breakfast	Snack	Lunch	Snack	Dinner	Snack	Bedtime	Night	Notes
Blood Sugar									
Insulin Dose									
Grams Carb									
Activity									

Date:	Breakfast	Snack	Lunch	Snack	Dinner	Snack	Bedtime	Night	Notes
Blood Sugar									
Insulin Dose									
Grams Carb									
Activity									

Date:	Breakfast	Snack	Lunch	Snack	Dinner	Snack	Bedtime	Night	Notes
Blood Sugar									
Insulin Dose									
Grams Carb									
Activity									

Weekly Diabetes Record

Name: ______________________________

Date:	Breakfast	Snack	Lunch	Snack	Dinner	Snack	Bedtime	Night	Notes
Blood Sugar									
Insulin Dose									
Grams Carb									
Activity									

Date:	Breakfast	Snack	Lunch	Snack	Dinner	Snack	Bedtime	Night	Notes
Blood Sugar									
Insulin Dose									
Grams Carb									
Activity									

Date:	Breakfast	Snack	Lunch	Snack	Dinner	Snack	Bedtime	Night	Notes
Blood Sugar									
Insulin Dose									
Grams Carb									
Activity									

Date:	Breakfast	Snack	Lunch	Snack	Dinner	Snack	Bedtime	Night	Notes
Blood Sugar									
Insulin Dose									
Grams Carb									
Activity									

Date:	Breakfast	Snack	Lunch	Snack	Dinner	Snack	Bedtime	Night	Notes
Blood Sugar									
Insulin Dose									
Grams Carb									
Activity									

Date:	Breakfast	Snack	Lunch	Snack	Dinner	Snack	Bedtime	Night	Notes
Blood Sugar									
Insulin Dose									
Grams Carb									
Activity									

Date:	Breakfast	Snack	Lunch	Snack	Dinner	Snack	Bedtime	Night	Notes
Blood Sugar									
Insulin Dose									
Grams Carb									
Activity									

Weekly Diabetes Record

Name: ____________________

Date:	Breakfast	Snack	Lunch	Snack	Dinner	Snack	Bedtime	Night	Notes
Blood Sugar									
Insulin Dose									
Grams Carb									
Activity									

Date:	Breakfast	Snack	Lunch	Snack	Dinner	Snack	Bedtime	Night	Notes
Blood Sugar									
Insulin Dose									
Grams Carb									
Activity									

Date:	Breakfast	Snack	Lunch	Snack	Dinner	Snack	Bedtime	Night	Notes
Blood Sugar									
Insulin Dose									
Grams Carb									
Activity									

Date:	Breakfast	Snack	Lunch	Snack	Dinner	Snack	Bedtime	Night	Notes
Blood Sugar									
Insulin Dose									
Grams Carb									
Activity									

Date:	Breakfast	Snack	Lunch	Snack	Dinner	Snack	Bedtime	Night	Notes
Blood Sugar									
Insulin Dose									
Grams Carb									
Activity									

Date:	Breakfast	Snack	Lunch	Snack	Dinner	Snack	Bedtime	Night	Notes
Blood Sugar									
Insulin Dose									
Grams Carb									
Activity									

Date:	Breakfast	Snack	Lunch	Snack	Dinner	Snack	Bedtime	Night	Notes
Blood Sugar									
Insulin Dose									
Grams Carb									
Activity									

Weekly Diabetes Record

Name: ______________________________

Date:	Breakfast	Snack	Lunch	Snack	Dinner	Snack	Bedtime	Night	Notes
Blood Sugar									
Insulin Dose									
Grams Carb									
Activity									

Date:	Breakfast	Snack	Lunch	Snack	Dinner	Snack	Bedtime	Night	Notes
Blood Sugar									
Insulin Dose									
Grams Carb									
Activity									

Date:	Breakfast	Snack	Lunch	Snack	Dinner	Snack	Bedtime	Night	Notes
Blood Sugar									
Insulin Dose									
Grams Carb									
Activity									

Date:	Breakfast	Snack	Lunch	Snack	Dinner	Snack	Bedtime	Night	Notes
Blood Sugar									
Insulin Dose									
Grams Carb									
Activity									

Date:	Breakfast	Snack	Lunch	Snack	Dinner	Snack	Bedtime	Night	Notes
Blood Sugar									
Insulin Dose									
Grams Carb									
Activity									

Date:	Breakfast	Snack	Lunch	Snack	Dinner	Snack	Bedtime	Night	Notes
Blood Sugar									
Insulin Dose									
Grams Carb									
Activity									

Date:	Breakfast	Snack	Lunch	Snack	Dinner	Snack	Bedtime	Night	Notes
Blood Sugar									
Insulin Dose									
Grams Carb									
Activity									

Weekly Diabetes Record

Name: ______________________________

Date:	Breakfast	Snack	Lunch	Snack	Dinner	Snack	Bedtime	Night	Notes
Blood Sugar									
Insulin Dose									
Grams Carb									
Activity									

Date:	Breakfast	Snack	Lunch	Snack	Dinner	Snack	Bedtime	Night	Notes
Blood Sugar									
Insulin Dose									
Grams Carb									
Activity									

Date:	Breakfast	Snack	Lunch	Snack	Dinner	Snack	Bedtime	Night	Notes
Blood Sugar									
Insulin Dose									
Grams Carb									
Activity									

Date:	Breakfast	Snack	Lunch	Snack	Dinner	Snack	Bedtime	Night	Notes
Blood Sugar									
Insulin Dose									
Grams Carb									
Activity									

Date:	Breakfast	Snack	Lunch	Snack	Dinner	Snack	Bedtime	Night	Notes
Blood Sugar									
Insulin Dose									
Grams Carb									
Activity									

Date:	Breakfast	Snack	Lunch	Snack	Dinner	Snack	Bedtime	Night	Notes
Blood Sugar									
Insulin Dose									
Grams Carb									
Activity									

Date:	Breakfast	Snack	Lunch	Snack	Dinner	Snack	Bedtime	Night	Notes
Blood Sugar									
Insulin Dose									
Grams Carb									
Activity									

Weekly Diabetes Record

Name: ______________________________

Date:	Breakfast	Snack	Lunch	Snack	Dinner	Snack	Bedtime	Night	Notes
Blood Sugar									
Insulin Dose									
Grams Carb									
Activity									

Date:	Breakfast	Snack	Lunch	Snack	Dinner	Snack	Bedtime	Night	Notes
Blood Sugar									
Insulin Dose									
Grams Carb									
Activity									

Date:	Breakfast	Snack	Lunch	Snack	Dinner	Snack	Bedtime	Night	Notes
Blood Sugar									
Insulin Dose									
Grams Carb									
Activity									

Date:	Breakfast	Snack	Lunch	Snack	Dinner	Snack	Bedtime	Night	Notes
Blood Sugar									
Insulin Dose									
Grams Carb									
Activity									

Date:	Breakfast	Snack	Lunch	Snack	Dinner	Snack	Bedtime	Night	Notes
Blood Sugar									
Insulin Dose									
Grams Carb									
Activity									

Date:	Breakfast	Snack	Lunch	Snack	Dinner	Snack	Bedtime	Night	Notes
Blood Sugar									
Insulin Dose									
Grams Carb									
Activity									

Date:	Breakfast	Snack	Lunch	Snack	Dinner	Snack	Bedtime	Night	Notes
Blood Sugar									
Insulin Dose									
Grams Carb									
Activity									

Weekly Diabetes Record

Name: ______________________________

Date:	Breakfast	Snack	Lunch	Snack	Dinner	Snack	Bedtime	Night	Notes
Blood Sugar									
Insulin Dose									
Grams Carb									
Activity									

Date:	Breakfast	Snack	Lunch	Snack	Dinner	Snack	Bedtime	Night	Notes
Blood Sugar									
Insulin Dose									
Grams Carb									
Activity									

Date:	Breakfast	Snack	Lunch	Snack	Dinner	Snack	Bedtime	Night	Notes
Blood Sugar									
Insulin Dose									
Grams Carb									
Activity									

Date:	Breakfast	Snack	Lunch	Snack	Dinner	Snack	Bedtime	Night	Notes
Blood Sugar									
Insulin Dose									
Grams Carb									
Activity									

Date:	Breakfast	Snack	Lunch	Snack	Dinner	Snack	Bedtime	Night	Notes
Blood Sugar									
Insulin Dose									
Grams Carb									
Activity									

Date:	Breakfast	Snack	Lunch	Snack	Dinner	Snack	Bedtime	Night	Notes
Blood Sugar									
Insulin Dose									
Grams Carb									
Activity									

Date:	Breakfast	Snack	Lunch	Snack	Dinner	Snack	Bedtime	Night	Notes
Blood Sugar									
Insulin Dose									
Grams Carb									
Activity									

Weekly Diabetes Record

Name: ______________________________

Date:	Breakfast	Snack	Lunch	Snack	Dinner	Snack	Bedtime	Night	Notes
Blood Sugar									
Insulin Dose									
Grams Carb									
Activity									

Date:	Breakfast	Snack	Lunch	Snack	Dinner	Snack	Bedtime	Night	Notes
Blood Sugar									
Insulin Dose									
Grams Carb									
Activity									

Date:	Breakfast	Snack	Lunch	Snack	Dinner	Snack	Bedtime	Night	Notes
Blood Sugar									
Insulin Dose									
Grams Carb									
Activity									

Date:	Breakfast	Snack	Lunch	Snack	Dinner	Snack	Bedtime	Night	Notes
Blood Sugar									
Insulin Dose									
Grams Carb									
Activity									

Date:	Breakfast	Snack	Lunch	Snack	Dinner	Snack	Bedtime	Night	Notes
Blood Sugar									
Insulin Dose									
Grams Carb									
Activity									

Date:	Breakfast	Snack	Lunch	Snack	Dinner	Snack	Bedtime	Night	Notes
Blood Sugar									
Insulin Dose									
Grams Carb									
Activity									

Date:	Breakfast	Snack	Lunch	Snack	Dinner	Snack	Bedtime	Night	Notes
Blood Sugar									
Insulin Dose									
Grams Carb									
Activity									

Weekly Diabetes Record

Name: ______________________________

Date:	Breakfast	Snack	Lunch	Snack	Dinner	Snack	Bedtime	Night	Notes
Blood Sugar									
Insulin Dose									
Grams Carb									
Activity									

Date:	Breakfast	Snack	Lunch	Snack	Dinner	Snack	Bedtime	Night	Notes
Blood Sugar									
Insulin Dose									
Grams Carb									
Activity									

Date:	Breakfast	Snack	Lunch	Snack	Dinner	Snack	Bedtime	Night	Notes
Blood Sugar									
Insulin Dose									
Grams Carb									
Activity									

Date:	Breakfast	Snack	Lunch	Snack	Dinner	Snack	Bedtime	Night	Notes
Blood Sugar									
Insulin Dose									
Grams Carb									
Activity									

Date:	Breakfast	Snack	Lunch	Snack	Dinner	Snack	Bedtime	Night	Notes
Blood Sugar									
Insulin Dose									
Grams Carb									
Activity									

Date:	Breakfast	Snack	Lunch	Snack	Dinner	Snack	Bedtime	Night	Notes
Blood Sugar									
Insulin Dose									
Grams Carb									
Activity									

Date:	Breakfast	Snack	Lunch	Snack	Dinner	Snack	Bedtime	Night	Notes
Blood Sugar									
Insulin Dose									
Grams Carb									
Activity									

Date:	Breakfast	Snack	Lunch	Snack	Dinner	Snack	Bedtime	Night	Notes
Blood Sugar									
Insulin Dose									
Grams Carb									
Activity									

Weekly Diabetes Record

Name: ______________________________

Date:	Breakfast	Snack	Lunch	Snack	Dinner	Snack	Bedtime	Night	Notes
Blood Sugar									
Insulin Dose									
Grams Carb									
Activity									

Date:	Breakfast	Snack	Lunch	Snack	Dinner	Snack	Bedtime	Night	Notes
Blood Sugar									
Insulin Dose									
Grams Carb									
Activity									

Date:	Breakfast	Snack	Lunch	Snack	Dinner	Snack	Bedtime	Night	Notes
Blood Sugar									
Insulin Dose									
Grams Carb									
Activity									

Date:	Breakfast	Snack	Lunch	Snack	Dinner	Snack	Bedtime	Night	Notes
Blood Sugar									
Insulin Dose									
Grams Carb									
Activity									

Date:	Breakfast	Snack	Lunch	Snack	Dinner	Snack	Bedtime	Night	Notes
Blood Sugar									
Insulin Dose									
Grams Carb									
Activity									

Date:	Breakfast	Snack	Lunch	Snack	Dinner	Snack	Bedtime	Night	Notes
Blood Sugar									
Insulin Dose									
Grams Carb									
Activity									

Date:	Breakfast	Snack	Lunch	Snack	Dinner	Snack	Bedtime	Night	Notes
Blood Sugar									
Insulin Dose									
Grams Carb									
Activity									

Weekly Diabetes Record

Name: ______________________________

Date:	Breakfast	Snack	Lunch	Snack	Dinner	Snack	Bedtime	Night	Notes
Blood Sugar									
Insulin Dose									
Grams Carb									
Activity									

Date:	Breakfast	Snack	Lunch	Snack	Dinner	Snack	Bedtime	Night	Notes
Blood Sugar									
Insulin Dose									
Grams Carb									
Activity									

Date:	Breakfast	Snack	Lunch	Snack	Dinner	Snack	Bedtime	Night	Notes
Blood Sugar									
Insulin Dose									
Grams Carb									
Activity									

Date:	Breakfast	Snack	Lunch	Snack	Dinner	Snack	Bedtime	Night	Notes
Blood Sugar									
Insulin Dose									
Grams Carb									
Activity									

Date:	Breakfast	Snack	Lunch	Snack	Dinner	Snack	Bedtime	Night	Notes
Blood Sugar									
Insulin Dose									
Grams Carb									
Activity									

Date:	Breakfast	Snack	Lunch	Snack	Dinner	Snack	Bedtime	Night	Notes
Blood Sugar									
Insulin Dose									
Grams Carb									
Activity									

Date:	Breakfast	Snack	Lunch	Snack	Dinner	Snack	Bedtime	Night	Notes
Blood Sugar									
Insulin Dose									
Grams Carb									
Activity									

Weekly Diabetes Record

Name: ____

Date:	Breakfast	Snack	Lunch	Snack	Dinner	Snack	Bedtime	Night	Notes
Blood Sugar									
Insulin Dose									
Grams Carb									
Activity									

Date:	Breakfast	Snack	Lunch	Snack	Dinner	Snack	Bedtime	Night	Notes
Blood Sugar									
Insulin Dose									
Grams Carb									
Activity									

Date:	Breakfast	Snack	Lunch	Snack	Dinner	Snack	Bedtime	Night	Notes
Blood Sugar									
Insulin Dose									
Grams Carb									
Activity									

Date:	Breakfast	Snack	Lunch	Snack	Dinner	Snack	Bedtime	Night	Notes
Blood Sugar									
Insulin Dose									
Grams Carb									
Activity									

Date:	Breakfast	Snack	Lunch	Snack	Dinner	Snack	Bedtime	Night	Notes
Blood Sugar									
Insulin Dose									
Grams Carb									
Activity									

Date:	Breakfast	Snack	Lunch	Snack	Dinner	Snack	Bedtime	Night	Notes
Blood Sugar									
Insulin Dose									
Grams Carb									
Activity									

Date:	Breakfast	Snack	Lunch	Snack	Dinner	Snack	Bedtime	Night	Notes
Blood Sugar									
Insulin Dose									
Grams Carb									
Activity									

Weekly Diabetes Record

Name: ______________________________

Date:	Breakfast	Snack	Lunch	Snack	Dinner	Snack	Bedtime	Night	Notes
Blood Sugar									
Insulin Dose									
Grams Carb									
Activity									

Date:	Breakfast	Snack	Lunch	Snack	Dinner	Snack	Bedtime	Night	Notes
Blood Sugar									
Insulin Dose									
Grams Carb									
Activity									

Date:	Breakfast	Snack	Lunch	Snack	Dinner	Snack	Bedtime	Night	Notes
Blood Sugar									
Insulin Dose									
Grams Carb									
Activity									

Date:	Breakfast	Snack	Lunch	Snack	Dinner	Snack	Bedtime	Night	Notes
Blood Sugar									
Insulin Dose									
Grams Carb									
Activity									

Date:	Breakfast	Snack	Lunch	Snack	Dinner	Snack	Bedtime	Night	Notes
Blood Sugar									
Insulin Dose									
Grams Carb									
Activity									

Date:	Breakfast	Snack	Lunch	Snack	Dinner	Snack	Bedtime	Night	Notes
Blood Sugar									
Insulin Dose									
Grams Carb									
Activity									

Date:	Breakfast	Snack	Lunch	Snack	Dinner	Snack	Bedtime	Night	Notes
Blood Sugar									
Insulin Dose									
Grams Carb									
Activity									

Weekly Diabetes Record

Name: ______________________________

Date:	Breakfast	Snack	Lunch	Snack	Dinner	Snack	Bedtime	Night	Notes
Blood Sugar									
Insulin Dose									
Grams Carb									
Activity									

Date:	Breakfast	Snack	Lunch	Snack	Dinner	Snack	Bedtime	Night	Notes
Blood Sugar									
Insulin Dose									
Grams Carb									
Activity									

Date:	Breakfast	Snack	Lunch	Snack	Dinner	Snack	Bedtime	Night	Notes
Blood Sugar									
Insulin Dose									
Grams Carb									
Activity									

Date:	Breakfast	Snack	Lunch	Snack	Dinner	Snack	Bedtime	Night	Notes
Blood Sugar									
Insulin Dose									
Grams Carb									
Activity									

Date:	Breakfast	Snack	Lunch	Snack	Dinner	Snack	Bedtime	Night	Notes
Blood Sugar									
Insulin Dose									
Grams Carb									
Activity									

Date:	Breakfast	Snack	Lunch	Snack	Dinner	Snack	Bedtime	Night	Notes
Blood Sugar									
Insulin Dose									
Grams Carb									
Activity									

Date:	Breakfast	Snack	Lunch	Snack	Dinner	Snack	Bedtime	Night	Notes
Blood Sugar									
Insulin Dose									
Grams Carb									
Activity									

Weekly Diabetes Record

Name: ______________________________

Date:	Breakfast	Snack	Lunch	Snack	Dinner	Snack	Bedtime	Night	Notes
Blood Sugar									
Insulin Dose									
Grams Carb									
Activity									

Date:	Breakfast	Snack	Lunch	Snack	Dinner	Snack	Bedtime	Night	Notes
Blood Sugar									
Insulin Dose									
Grams Carb									
Activity									

Date:	Breakfast	Snack	Lunch	Snack	Dinner	Snack	Bedtime	Night	Notes
Blood Sugar									
Insulin Dose									
Grams Carb									
Activity									

Date:	Breakfast	Snack	Lunch	Snack	Dinner	Snack	Bedtime	Night	Notes
Blood Sugar									
Insulin Dose									
Grams Carb									
Activity									

Date:	Breakfast	Snack	Lunch	Snack	Dinner	Snack	Bedtime	Night	Notes
Blood Sugar									
Insulin Dose									
Grams Carb									
Activity									

Date:	Breakfast	Snack	Lunch	Snack	Dinner	Snack	Bedtime	Night	Notes
Blood Sugar									
Insulin Dose									
Grams Carb									
Activity									

Date:	Breakfast	Snack	Lunch	Snack	Dinner	Snack	Bedtime	Night	Notes
Blood Sugar									
Insulin Dose									
Grams Carb									
Activity									

Weekly Diabetes Record

Name: ______________________________

Date:	Breakfast	Snack	Lunch	Snack	Dinner	Snack	Bedtime	Night	Notes
Blood Sugar									
Insulin Dose									
Grams Carb									
Activity									

Date:	Breakfast	Snack	Lunch	Snack	Dinner	Snack	Bedtime	Night	Notes
Blood Sugar									
Insulin Dose									
Grams Carb									
Activity									

Date:	Breakfast	Snack	Lunch	Snack	Dinner	Snack	Bedtime	Night	Notes
Blood Sugar									
Insulin Dose									
Grams Carb									
Activity									

Date:	Breakfast	Snack	Lunch	Snack	Dinner	Snack	Bedtime	Night	Notes
Blood Sugar									
Insulin Dose									
Grams Carb									
Activity									

Date:	Breakfast	Snack	Lunch	Snack	Dinner	Snack	Bedtime	Night	Notes
Blood Sugar									
Insulin Dose									
Grams Carb									
Activity									

Date:	Breakfast	Snack	Lunch	Snack	Dinner	Snack	Bedtime	Night	Notes
Blood Sugar									
Insulin Dose									
Grams Carb									
Activity									

Date:	Breakfast	Snack	Lunch	Snack	Dinner	Snack	Bedtime	Night	Notes
Blood Sugar									
Insulin Dose									
Grams Carb									
Activity									

Weekly Diabetes Record

Name: ______________________________

Date:	Breakfast	Snack	Lunch	Snack	Dinner	Snack	Bedtime	Night	Notes
Blood Sugar									
Insulin Dose									
Grams Carb									
Activity									

Date:	Breakfast	Snack	Lunch	Snack	Dinner	Snack	Bedtime	Night	Notes
Blood Sugar									
Insulin Dose									
Grams Carb									
Activity									

Date:	Breakfast	Snack	Lunch	Snack	Dinner	Snack	Bedtime	Night	Notes
Blood Sugar									
Insulin Dose									
Grams Carb									
Activity									

Date:	Breakfast	Snack	Lunch	Snack	Dinner	Snack	Bedtime	Night	Notes
Blood Sugar									
Insulin Dose									
Grams Carb									
Activity									

Date:	Breakfast	Snack	Lunch	Snack	Dinner	Snack	Bedtime	Night	Notes
Blood Sugar									
Insulin Dose									
Grams Carb									
Activity									

Date:	Breakfast	Snack	Lunch	Snack	Dinner	Snack	Bedtime	Night	Notes
Blood Sugar									
Insulin Dose									
Grams Carb									
Activity									

Date:	Breakfast	Snack	Lunch	Snack	Dinner	Snack	Bedtime	Night	Notes
Blood Sugar									
Insulin Dose									
Grams Carb									
Activity									

Weekly Diabetes Record

Name: ______________________________

Date:	Breakfast	Snack	Lunch	Snack	Dinner	Snack	Bedtime	Night	Notes
Blood Sugar									
Insulin Dose									
Grams Carb									
Activity									

Date:	Breakfast	Snack	Lunch	Snack	Dinner	Snack	Bedtime	Night	Notes
Blood Sugar									
Insulin Dose									
Grams Carb									
Activity									

Date:	Breakfast	Snack	Lunch	Snack	Dinner	Snack	Bedtime	Night	Notes
Blood Sugar									
Insulin Dose									
Grams Carb									
Activity									

Date:	Breakfast	Snack	Lunch	Snack	Dinner	Snack	Bedtime	Night	Notes
Blood Sugar									
Insulin Dose									
Grams Carb									
Activity									

Date:	Breakfast	Snack	Lunch	Snack	Dinner	Snack	Bedtime	Night	Notes
Blood Sugar									
Insulin Dose									
Grams Carb									
Activity									

Date:	Breakfast	Snack	Lunch	Snack	Dinner	Snack	Bedtime	Night	Notes
Blood Sugar									
Insulin Dose									
Grams Carb									
Activity									

Date:	Breakfast	Snack	Lunch	Snack	Dinner	Snack	Bedtime	Night	Notes
Blood Sugar									
Insulin Dose									
Grams Carb									
Activity									

Weekly Diabetes Record

Name: ______________________________

Date:	Breakfast	Snack	Lunch	Snack	Dinner	Snack	Bedtime	Night	Notes
Blood Sugar									
Insulin Dose									
Grams Carb									
Activity									

Date:	Breakfast	Snack	Lunch	Snack	Dinner	Snack	Bedtime	Night	Notes
Blood Sugar									
Insulin Dose									
Grams Carb									
Activity									

Date:	Breakfast	Snack	Lunch	Snack	Dinner	Snack	Bedtime	Night	Notes
Blood Sugar									
Insulin Dose									
Grams Carb									
Activity									

Date:	Breakfast	Snack	Lunch	Snack	Dinner	Snack	Bedtime	Night	Notes
Blood Sugar									
Insulin Dose									
Grams Carb									
Activity									

Date:	Breakfast	Snack	Lunch	Snack	Dinner	Snack	Bedtime	Night	Notes
Blood Sugar									
Insulin Dose									
Grams Carb									
Activity									

Date:	Breakfast	Snack	Lunch	Snack	Dinner	Snack	Bedtime	Night	Notes
Blood Sugar									
Insulin Dose									
Grams Carb									
Activity									

Date:	Breakfast	Snack	Lunch	Snack	Dinner	Snack	Bedtime	Night	Notes
Blood Sugar									
Insulin Dose									
Grams Carb									
Activity									

Weekly Diabetes Record

Name: ________________________________

Date:	Breakfast	Snack	Lunch	Snack	Dinner	Snack	Bedtime	Night	Notes
Blood Sugar									
Insulin Dose									
Grams Carb									
Activity									

Date:	Breakfast	Snack	Lunch	Snack	Dinner	Snack	Bedtime	Night	Notes
Blood Sugar									
Insulin Dose									
Grams Carb									
Activity									

Date:	Breakfast	Snack	Lunch	Snack	Dinner	Snack	Bedtime	Night	Notes
Blood Sugar									
Insulin Dose									
Grams Carb									
Activity									

Date:	Breakfast	Snack	Lunch	Snack	Dinner	Snack	Bedtime	Night	Notes
Blood Sugar									
Insulin Dose									
Grams Carb									
Activity									

Date:	Breakfast	Snack	Lunch	Snack	Dinner	Snack	Bedtime	Night	Notes
Blood Sugar									
Insulin Dose									
Grams Carb									
Activity									

Date:	Breakfast	Snack	Lunch	Snack	Dinner	Snack	Bedtime	Night	Notes
Blood Sugar									
Insulin Dose									
Grams Carb									
Activity									

Date:	Breakfast	Snack	Lunch	Snack	Dinner	Snack	Bedtime	Night	Notes
Blood Sugar									
Insulin Dose									
Grams Carb									
Activity									

Weekly Diabetes Record

Name: ______________________________

Date:	Breakfast	Snack	Lunch	Snack	Dinner	Snack	Bedtime	Night	Notes
Blood Sugar									
Insulin Dose									
Grams Carb									
Activity									

Date:	Breakfast	Snack	Lunch	Snack	Dinner	Snack	Bedtime	Night	Notes
Blood Sugar									
Insulin Dose									
Grams Carb									
Activity									

Date:	Breakfast	Snack	Lunch	Snack	Dinner	Snack	Bedtime	Night	Notes
Blood Sugar									
Insulin Dose									
Grams Carb									
Activity									

Date:	Breakfast	Snack	Lunch	Snack	Dinner	Snack	Bedtime	Night	Notes
Blood Sugar									
Insulin Dose									
Grams Carb									
Activity									

Date:	Breakfast	Snack	Lunch	Snack	Dinner	Snack	Bedtime	Night	Notes
Blood Sugar									
Insulin Dose									
Grams Carb									
Activity									

Date:	Breakfast	Snack	Lunch	Snack	Dinner	Snack	Bedtime	Night	Notes
Blood Sugar									
Insulin Dose									
Grams Carb									
Activity									

Date:	Breakfast	Snack	Lunch	Snack	Dinner	Snack	Bedtime	Night	Notes
Blood Sugar									
Insulin Dose									
Grams Carb									
Activity									

Weekly Diabetes Record

Name: ____

Date:	Breakfast	Snack	Lunch	Snack	Dinner	Snack	Bedtime	Night	Notes
Blood Sugar									
Insulin Dose									
Grams Carb									
Activity									

Date:	Breakfast	Snack	Lunch	Snack	Dinner	Snack	Bedtime	Night	Notes
Blood Sugar									
Insulin Dose									
Grams Carb									
Activity									

Date:	Breakfast	Snack	Lunch	Snack	Dinner	Snack	Bedtime	Night	Notes
Blood Sugar									
Insulin Dose									
Grams Carb									
Activity									

Date:	Breakfast	Snack	Lunch	Snack	Dinner	Snack	Bedtime	Night	Notes
Blood Sugar									
Insulin Dose									
Grams Carb									
Activity									

Date:	Breakfast	Snack	Lunch	Snack	Dinner	Snack	Bedtime	Night	Notes
Blood Sugar									
Insulin Dose									
Grams Carb									
Activity									

Date:	Breakfast	Snack	Lunch	Snack	Dinner	Snack	Bedtime	Night	Notes
Blood Sugar									
Insulin Dose									
Grams Carb									
Activity									

Date:	Breakfast	Snack	Lunch	Snack	Dinner	Snack	Bedtime	Night	Notes
Blood Sugar									
Insulin Dose									
Grams Carb									
Activity									

Weekly Diabetes Record

Name: ______________________________

Date:	Breakfast	Snack	Lunch	Snack	Dinner	Snack	Bedtime	Night	Notes
Blood Sugar									
Insulin Dose									
Grams Carb									
Activity									

Date:	Breakfast	Snack	Lunch	Snack	Dinner	Snack	Bedtime	Night	Notes
Blood Sugar									
Insulin Dose									
Grams Carb									
Activity									

Date:	Breakfast	Snack	Lunch	Snack	Dinner	Snack	Bedtime	Night	Notes
Blood Sugar									
Insulin Dose									
Grams Carb									
Activity									

Date:	Breakfast	Snack	Lunch	Snack	Dinner	Snack	Bedtime	Night	Notes
Blood Sugar									
Insulin Dose									
Grams Carb									
Activity									

Date:	Breakfast	Snack	Lunch	Snack	Dinner	Snack	Bedtime	Night	Notes
Blood Sugar									
Insulin Dose									
Grams Carb									
Activity									

Date:	Breakfast	Snack	Lunch	Snack	Dinner	Snack	Bedtime	Night	Notes
Blood Sugar									
Insulin Dose									
Grams Carb									
Activity									

Date:	Breakfast	Snack	Lunch	Snack	Dinner	Snack	Bedtime	Night	Notes
Blood Sugar									
Insulin Dose									
Grams Carb									
Activity									

Weekly Diabetes Record

Name: ____

Date:	Breakfast	Snack	Lunch	Snack	Dinner	Snack	Bedtime	Night	Notes
Blood Sugar									
Insulin Dose									
Grams Carb									
Activity									

Date:	Breakfast	Snack	Lunch	Snack	Dinner	Snack	Bedtime	Night	Notes
Blood Sugar									
Insulin Dose									
Grams Carb									
Activity									

Date:	Breakfast	Snack	Lunch	Snack	Dinner	Snack	Bedtime	Night	Notes
Blood Sugar									
Insulin Dose									
Grams Carb									
Activity									

Date:	Breakfast	Snack	Lunch	Snack	Dinner	Snack	Bedtime	Night	Notes
Blood Sugar									
Insulin Dose									
Grams Carb									
Activity									

Date:	Breakfast	Snack	Lunch	Snack	Dinner	Snack	Bedtime	Night	Notes
Blood Sugar									
Insulin Dose									
Grams Carb									
Activity									

Date:	Breakfast	Snack	Lunch	Snack	Dinner	Snack	Bedtime	Night	Notes
Blood Sugar									
Insulin Dose									
Grams Carb									
Activity									

Date:	Breakfast	Snack	Lunch	Snack	Dinner	Snack	Bedtime	Night	Notes
Blood Sugar									
Insulin Dose									
Grams Carb									
Activity									

Weekly Diabetes Record

Name: ______________________________

Date:	Breakfast	Snack	Lunch	Snack	Dinner	Snack	Bedtime	Night	Notes
Blood Sugar									
Insulin Dose									
Grams Carb									
Activity									

Date:	Breakfast	Snack	Lunch	Snack	Dinner	Snack	Bedtime	Night	Notes
Blood Sugar									
Insulin Dose									
Grams Carb									
Activity									

Date:	Breakfast	Snack	Lunch	Snack	Dinner	Snack	Bedtime	Night	Notes
Blood Sugar									
Insulin Dose									
Grams Carb									
Activity									

Date:	Breakfast	Snack	Lunch	Snack	Dinner	Snack	Bedtime	Night	Notes
Blood Sugar									
Insulin Dose									
Grams Carb									
Activity									

Date:	Breakfast	Snack	Lunch	Snack	Dinner	Snack	Bedtime	Night	Notes
Blood Sugar									
Insulin Dose									
Grams Carb									
Activity									

Date:	Breakfast	Snack	Lunch	Snack	Dinner	Snack	Bedtime	Night	Notes
Blood Sugar									
Insulin Dose									
Grams Carb									
Activity									

Date:	Breakfast	Snack	Lunch	Snack	Dinner	Snack	Bedtime	Night	Notes
Blood Sugar									
Insulin Dose									
Grams Carb									
Activity									

Weekly Diabetes Record

Name: ______________________________

Date:	Breakfast	Snack	Lunch	Snack	Dinner	Snack	Bedtime	Night	Notes
Blood Sugar									
Insulin Dose									
Grams Carb									
Activity									

Date:	Breakfast	Snack	Lunch	Snack	Dinner	Snack	Bedtime	Night	Notes
Blood Sugar									
Insulin Dose									
Grams Carb									
Activity									

Date:	Breakfast	Snack	Lunch	Snack	Dinner	Snack	Bedtime	Night	Notes
Blood Sugar									
Insulin Dose									
Grams Carb									
Activity									

Date:	Breakfast	Snack	Lunch	Snack	Dinner	Snack	Bedtime	Night	Notes
Blood Sugar									
Insulin Dose									
Grams Carb									
Activity									

Date:	Breakfast	Snack	Lunch	Snack	Dinner	Snack	Bedtime	Night	Notes
Blood Sugar									
Insulin Dose									
Grams Carb									
Activity									

Date:	Breakfast	Snack	Lunch	Snack	Dinner	Snack	Bedtime	Night	Notes
Blood Sugar									
Insulin Dose									
Grams Carb									
Activity									

Date:	Breakfast	Snack	Lunch	Snack	Dinner	Snack	Bedtime	Night	Notes
Blood Sugar									
Insulin Dose									
Grams Carb									
Activity									

Weekly Diabetes Record

Name: ______________________________

Date:	Breakfast	Snack	Lunch	Snack	Dinner	Snack	Bedtime	Night	Notes
Blood Sugar									
Insulin Dose									
Grams Carb									
Activity									

Date:	Breakfast	Snack	Lunch	Snack	Dinner	Snack	Bedtime	Night	Notes
Blood Sugar									
Insulin Dose									
Grams Carb									
Activity									

Date:	Breakfast	Snack	Lunch	Snack	Dinner	Snack	Bedtime	Night	Notes
Blood Sugar									
Insulin Dose									
Grams Carb									
Activity									

Date:	Breakfast	Snack	Lunch	Snack	Dinner	Snack	Bedtime	Night	Notes
Blood Sugar									
Insulin Dose									
Grams Carb									
Activity									

Date:	Breakfast	Snack	Lunch	Snack	Dinner	Snack	Bedtime	Night	Notes
Blood Sugar									
Insulin Dose									
Grams Carb									
Activity									

Date:	Breakfast	Snack	Lunch	Snack	Dinner	Snack	Bedtime	Night	Notes
Blood Sugar									
Insulin Dose									
Grams Carb									
Activity									

Date:	Breakfast	Snack	Lunch	Snack	Dinner	Snack	Bedtime	Night	Notes
Blood Sugar									
Insulin Dose									
Grams Carb									
Activity									

Weekly Diabetes Record

Name: ______________________________

Date:	Breakfast	Snack	Lunch	Snack	Dinner	Snack	Bedtime	Night	Notes
Blood Sugar									
Insulin Dose									
Grams Carb									
Activity									

Date:	Breakfast	Snack	Lunch	Snack	Dinner	Snack	Bedtime	Night	Notes
Blood Sugar									
Insulin Dose									
Grams Carb									
Activity									

Date:	Breakfast	Snack	Lunch	Snack	Dinner	Snack	Bedtime	Night	Notes
Blood Sugar									
Insulin Dose									
Grams Carb									
Activity									

Date:	Breakfast	Snack	Lunch	Snack	Dinner	Snack	Bedtime	Night	Notes
Blood Sugar									
Insulin Dose									
Grams Carb									
Activity									

Date:	Breakfast	Snack	Lunch	Snack	Dinner	Snack	Bedtime	Night	Notes
Blood Sugar									
Insulin Dose									
Grams Carb									
Activity									

Date:	Breakfast	Snack	Lunch	Snack	Dinner	Snack	Bedtime	Night	Notes
Blood Sugar									
Insulin Dose									
Grams Carb									
Activity									

Date:	Breakfast	Snack	Lunch	Snack	Dinner	Snack	Bedtime	Night	Notes
Blood Sugar									
Insulin Dose									
Grams Carb									
Activity									

Weekly Diabetes Record

Name: ______________________________

Date:	Breakfast	Snack	Lunch	Snack	Dinner	Snack	Bedtime	Night	Notes
Blood Sugar									
Insulin Dose									
Grams Carb									
Activity									

Date:	Breakfast	Snack	Lunch	Snack	Dinner	Snack	Bedtime	Night	Notes
Blood Sugar									
Insulin Dose									
Grams Carb									
Activity									

Date:	Breakfast	Snack	Lunch	Snack	Dinner	Snack	Bedtime	Night	Notes
Blood Sugar									
Insulin Dose									
Grams Carb									
Activity									

Date:	Breakfast	Snack	Lunch	Snack	Dinner	Snack	Bedtime	Night	Notes
Blood Sugar									
Insulin Dose									
Grams Carb									
Activity									

Date:	Breakfast	Snack	Lunch	Snack	Dinner	Snack	Bedtime	Night	Notes
Blood Sugar									
Insulin Dose									
Grams Carb									
Activity									

Date:	Breakfast	Snack	Lunch	Snack	Dinner	Snack	Bedtime	Night	Notes
Blood Sugar									
Insulin Dose									
Grams Carb									
Activity									

Date:	Breakfast	Snack	Lunch	Snack	Dinner	Snack	Bedtime	Night	Notes
Blood Sugar									
Insulin Dose									
Grams Carb									
Activity									

Made in the USA
Las Vegas, NV
23 January 2021

16437387R00111